ACID REFLUX IN CHILDREN

ACID REFLUX IN CHILDREN

How Healthy Eating Can Fix Your Child's Asthma,
Allergies, Obesity, Nasal Congestion, Cough & Croup

A Parent's Guide to Reflux in Infants, Children & Teens

Jamie Koufman, M.D, F.A.C.S.

New York Times Bestselling Author of *Dropping Acid: The Reflux Diet Cookbook & Cure*

Julie L. Wei, M.D. & Karen B. Zur, M.D.

Katalitix Media, New York

NOTICE AND DISCLAIMER
This book is intended as a reference volume only, not as a medical manual. The information given here is designed to help you make informed decisions about your family's eating habits. It is not intended as a substitute for any treatment that might have been prescribed by a physician. If you suspect that you or your child has a medical problem, we urge you to seek medical help. Any use of this book is at the reader's discretion, as the advice and strategies contained within may not be suitable for every individual.

The opinions of the authors expressed in this book are based upon their research and clinical experience. The authors do not claim to have reviewed all of the scientific data on reflux, nutrition, and the American diet, and recognize (and disclose) that there are divergent opinions about the topics and recommendations presented herein.

Cover photo by iStock/JBRyson

ISBN: 978-1-940561-05-9
EBOOK ISBN: 978-1-940561-06-6

To our patients and to the millions of children
whose unhealthy diets can and must be fixed

CONTENTS

PART I

UNDERSTANDING REFLUX IN CHILDREN

PART II

RECIPES FOR REFLUX REPAIR

Paradigm Shift:
Bad Food Causes Acid Reflux
and Respiratory Disease

"No disease that can be treated with diet should be
treated by any other means." —Maimonides

Acid Reflux in Children: How Healthy Eating Can Fix Your Child's Asthma, Allergies, Obesity, Nasal Congestion, Cough & Croup is a profoundly important book. It's bad enough that acid reflux affects so many adults; that it afflicts tens of millions of children represents a massive and shocking public health problem that must be acknowledged and addressed. And, for children, a diet filled with processed food, fast food, and sweet soft drinks has consequences beyond reflux, as demonstrated by alarmingly high and ever-increasing rates of childhood obesity and diabetes. It's time that we take a responsible look at our children's diets.

As a gastroenterologist specializing in acid reflux for thirty years, I have witnessed remarkable changes in how we understand and approach this disease. Initially, gastroenterologists learned to improve patients' symptoms of heartburn without actually controlling the underlying disease. On our strongest anti-reflux medications, patients still continued to have reflux; over time, it has become clear that medication alone is *not* the silver bullet we had once hoped it to be.

Thanks, in large measure, to the work of my friend and colleague, Dr. Jamie Koufman, "respiratory reflux" has exploded onto the scene, *and* we have come to recognize the central role played by the unhealthy American diet in causing it. In the time I have known Dr. Koufman, she has devoted herself to changing the mindset of both physicians and the public, stressing that medications (i.e., "purple pills") are not the answer. She has taught us that diet and lifestyle changes are crucial for effective reflux management and cure. For many clinicians who treat reflux, this strategy has been, and continues to be, a game-changer. We now understand that respiratory reflux is the most common cause of "allergies," "asthma," chronic cough, too much throat mucus, chronic throat-clearing, hoarseness, sore throat, shortness of breath, and even many lung diseases.

Acid Reflux in Children: How Healthy Eating Can Fix Your Child's Asthma, Allergies, Obesity, Nasal Congestion, Cough & Croup needs to be read by all who care about our children's health and well-being. I recommend this book not just to parents but also to pediatricians, otolaryngologists, allergists, pulmonologists—and yes, we gastroenterologists, too.

David M. Gutman, M.D., F.A.C.G. (Gastroenterologist)
Director, Reflux Program of the North Shore University
Hospital Zucker School of Medicine at Hofstra
Northwell Health, Long Island, New York

The Respiratory Reflux Revolution

Every year, tens of millions of infants, children, and teens are misdiagnosed as having asthma, allergies, nasal congestion, ear infections, chronic cough, breathing problems, and croup when the real problem is, in fact, acid reflux.

Reflux is the great masquerader of our time, and as you will learn, reflux has many aliases, confusing parents and doctors alike and leading to improper treatment and continued suffering for children. Just take a look at the myriad symptoms that acid reflux is responsible for:

Spitting up	Ear infections
Difficulty feeding	Fluid in ears
Interrupted sleep	Raspy voice
Poor sleeping	Weak voice
Chronic cough	Allergies
Recurrent croup	Always has a "cold"
Noisy breathing	Asthma
Pneumonia	Sore throat
Shortness of breath	Overweight
Choking episodes	Obesity
Nasal congestion	Snoring
Runny nose	Eczema
Too much mucus	Laryngomalacia
Chronic throat-clearing	Glottic stenosis
Difficulty swallowing	Sinus infections
Throwing up	Subglottic stenosis

All of the above symptoms and conditions can be *caused or made worse* by acid reflux; indeed, those listed are among the most common misdiagnoses in America. In other words, stuffy nose, allergies, asthma, croup, and chronic cough may, in fact, be fixed by anti-reflux treatment in the absence of any medical intervention.[1-5]*

Unlike adults who may have obvious reflux symptoms (indigestion and heartburn, for example), children are almost always "silent refluxers," silent because children with reflux rarely complain of heartburn or indigestion, which makes reflux mysterious, difficult to diagnose, and easy to overlook. See the quizzes on pages 12–13 to discover if your child has acid reflux or is at high risk because of a "bad reflux diet."

Respiratory Reflux Is the Missing Link

Respiratory reflux is the missing link between misdiagnosed "allergies," "sinusitis," and "asthma," and the underlying cause, acid reflux, which can be successfully managed with a healthy diet and lifestyle.

But there is good news! Once reflux is identified or even suspected, the fix is more in your control than you may think. I have devoted my career to advancing the field of respiratory reflux,[4,6] that is, acid reflux that causes ear, nose, throat, and voice problems, as well as serious lung problems, including asthma, chronic bronchitis, and cough.[3] Traditionally, reflux has been associated mainly with the GI tract, but I have found that acid reflux may affect any and all parts of the respiratory tract, too, with insidious effects that are costing our kids their health. "Respiratory reflux" is a relatively new term I coined to bring attention to the fact that acid reflux can cause respiratory disease.[4,6] It is intended to replace older medical terms such as airway reflux, extraesophageal reflux, and laryngopharyngeal reflux (LPR) as a more accurate and intuitive term that people seem to readily understand.

Reflux in children is poorly understood, even by pediatricians and other medical specialists. Today, respiratory reflux hides in plain sight. For example, your pediatrician or even a specialist might have told you that your child has asthma, sinusitis, or allergy, when, in fact, s/he has reflux. Perhaps even your doctor prescribed an antacid medication, which had no beneficial effects.

*See references, p. 226.

The real villain, however, is not vanquished merely by pills. Most medications by themselves won't do a thing for most children's reflux symptoms. Why should you care? Because reflux is not only uncomfortable and inconvenient, it's dangerous. If left improperly treated, or untreated, reflux can wreak havoc on your child's ears, nose, throat, airways, lungs, and digestive system. If left misdiagnosed, the improper use of medications can also be detrimental to your child's health.

"Why didn't my doctor know about this?" you might ask. Part of the problem is that doctors are too specialized. The go-to reflux doctor, the gastrointestinal specialist (GI), is focused on the swallowing tube (esophagus) and stomach, but most often doesn't recognize that a child can have respiratory reflux without having any esophageal or stomach symptoms.

To make matters worse, allergists, ENTs (ear, nose, and throat doctors), and lung doctors (pulmonologists) rely on GIs to diagnose reflux, but GI doctors have no way to diagnose respiratory reflux because they're not looking at the right area of the body. Indeed, the fragmentation of the medical specialties is such that when it comes to respiratory reflux, most doctors cannot see the forest for the trees. Furthermore, reflux in children is rarely a "medical condition," because reflux with all its complications is a consequence of what and when your child eats. At its core, it's about fixing your child's diet.

Take a look at our letter to physicians on page xvi. It is a call to action for all doctors to consider diet first before writing a prescription. I adhere to the teachings of Hippocrates: "Let food be thy medicine and medicine be thy food," especially in the case of children.

In the past sixty years, the diet of most Americans has changed for the worse,[1-5,7-18] and there has been no captain steering the ship—no overarching body to monitor all aspects of the safety of the food we eat. Instead of protecting the public, the Food and Drug Administration and the U.S. Department of Agriculture have primarily served the financial interests of the food industry. That means dubious practices like accepting money from "sponsors," who make the food that is ultimately making your child sick. And it's not just the FDA and the USDA. It's the American Diabetes Association, the American Heart Association, and many of the other governing bodies that are supposed to be keeping us healthy and informed.[1,14-16]

The reflux conundrum helps explain why many reflux-related diseases are on the rise in America—affecting approximately half of all Americans.[2]

Today, excessive amounts of acid and other harmful chemicals are found in virtually everything packaged in bottles and cans.[1] An astounding 75 to 80 percent of all goods in the grocery store aisle have sugar added and contain excessive quantities of fat, both leading causes of acid reflux.[1,2,4] Most food in the supermarket really isn't food at all.

As an ear, nose, and throat physician, I have learned most of what I know about reflux from my patients. Over years of practice, I've seen the correlation between patients eliminating certain foods and the eradication of their chronic symptoms (many of whom were initially misdiagnosed as requiring extensive testing, harmful medications, or even surgery). And after forty years of doctoring, I am quite certain that the key to wellness and vanquishing acid reflux is healthy diet and lifestyle—period! With proper intervention, even my sickest patients who suffer from bad breathing and damaged lungs can recover.

I have, frankly, become tired of hearing stories of children being carted off to specialists for no reason or given harmful steroids for a misdiagnosed "allergy" or "asthma." Too many unnecessary surgeries are performed on toddlers for ear tubes and tonsillitis. I've heard righteous indignation from parents, who say, "It's one thing for me to be fooled by the food industry, but it's another to be misled by doctors—I need to do better for my child."

Here's something to consider: tonsillitis, sinusitis, and every other "itis" your child is diagnosed with simply means that that area of the body is inflamed. Guess what most commonly causes inflammation in these parts of the body? Reflux.

While the fix is more in your control than you may think, it's not always simple. It isn't easy to change one's habitual eating habits, preferences, schedules, and patterns of dietary behavior. I tell parents that a successful reflux rehabilitation program is a platform for change with the long-term goal of health maintenance and disease prevention for the whole family. For overweight children, the greatest side benefit of our reflux program is that they lose weight naturally and slowly with a diet that is simply "lean, clean, green, and alkaline."

When I fix a child's reflux, the knowledge imparted to the parents translates to significant dietary changes for the whole family. My experience with young parents was a major impetus for this book, but in order to tell the complete story, I knew that I needed to seek out coauthors with both a passion and knowledge of pediatrics.

Lightning strikes! Dr. Julie Wei and Dr. Karen Zur, both pediatric ENT experts, share my views about the importance of diet and lifestyle in treating reflux and health in general. This book represents a true collaborative effort. Every word expresses all three of our voices, including in total almost one hundred years of combined clinical experience.

We believe that this seminal book will help change how America eats, how doctors diagnose and treat, and most importantly, allow our needlessly sick children and grandchildren to live healthier, more fulfilling lives.

Here's to our future—healthy children.

Jamie Koufman, M.D., F.A.C.S.
Director, Voice Institute of New York, Clinical Professor
of Otolaryngology, New York Eye and Ear Infirmary of the
Mount Sinai Medical System, New York, New York

An Open Letter to Physicians

(Parents, You'll Want to Check This Out Too)

Dear Colleague:

Most babies are born healthy, and within two years, most children are sick. Chronic rhinorrhea (runny nose) and nasal congestion are often diagnosed as "allergy" or "sinusitis," while breathing problems are commonly attributed to "asthma." We use quotes around these diagnoses, because it is our experience that children are frequently misdiagnosed and do not suffer from allergy or asthma at all. Ear infections and other breathing problems are, likewise, caused and exacerbated by factors that are completely controllable and preventable.

In the experience of the authors, physicians often overlook and underplay the pernicious effects of an unhealthy diet and acid reflux. The fact of the matter is that unhealthy diets and lifestyles wreak havoc on our children's health, and physicians who continue to overlook the role of diet in disease—causation, treatment, and prevention—are doing a major disservice to their patients.

This book is dedicated to the premise that nutrition and lifestyle changes are imperative for better health for the entire family, beginning in infancy. What we have shared with parents in this book thus far is Dr. Jamie's explanation of respiratory reflux.[4,6] Respiratory reflux is real, and we believe it is responsible for as much as seventy percent of respiratory diseases.

What is respiratory reflux? It is acid reflux into the nose, throat, trachea, bronchi, and lungs, also known as extraesophageal reflux or laryngopharyngeal reflux (LPR). Eavesdrop on your local playground and you will undoubtedly hear how the symptoms of this type of acid reflux are ubiquitous. Too often parents aren't complaining specifically about respiratory reflux: they're sharing details on inhalers and steroids, antibiotics and testing, possible surgery for adenoids and ear tubes, and referrals to specialists like otolaryngologists and pulmonologists—treatments for problems stemming from respiratory reflux. These treatments are unnecessary, but only if reflux is detected and addressed appropriately.

We believe that physicians, especially pediatricians and allergists, should consider the diet of their sick patients first and foremost as the cause of underlying respiratory reflux before pursuing alternative diagnoses and treatments. Most do not. Too many times, we've treated children who have seen several doctors before us, only to discover they have been misinformed, misdiagnosed, and mistreated when their problem was as simple as a bad diet.[1-5, 7-18]

Respiratory reflux is prevalent, and it can cause, exacerbate, or complicate any and all respiratory diseases. In infants and children, reflux can be linked to ear infections, sinus disease, laryngomalacia, glottic stenosis and subglottic stenosis, and other serious airway problems. In most cases neither H2-antagonists nor proton pump inhibitors control respiratory reflux. The root causes must be addressed.

From the Case Files of Dr. Jamie:
Relapsing Polychondritis & Respiratory Reflux

In 2000, William, a previously healthy teenager, presented with a tracheotomy in place (for two years) and a diagnosis of aggressive relapsing polychondritis, a rare, idiopathic autoimmune disease that attacks cartilage, particularly the cartilage of the ears, nose, and airway (larynx and trachea). His medical care was being managed at two famous academic medical centers, both of which told the patient and his family that William had a relentless disease and might die. One institution was contemplating a stem cell transplant.

In my experience, relapsing polychondritis is usually a slow, indolent disease. I had never seen an aggressively progressive case. After examining the patient's laryngopharynx, I concluded that he might have acid reflux as an "accelerant." Reflux testing (pharyngeal pH-monitoring) confirmed severe reflux and medical anti-reflux treatment was initiated. Two months later, repeat pH-monitoring revealed medical treatment was failing, so I initiated a fundoplication. The anti-reflux surgery was subsequently performed, and almost miraculously, three months after the surgery, I was able to remove William's tracheotomy. Today, William is a thirty-five-year-old married man with children. He runs a successful business, and his relapsing polychondritis is stable.

The above case is exemplary of the interaction between two inflammatory diseases simultaneously affecting the airway. The impact of reflux on coexistent respiratory diseases cannot be overestimated.

Since the 1960s, the American diet has changed dramatically for the worse, and it bears responsibility for a large proportion of respiratory disease in children. Not only can respiratory reflux cause symptoms, it can exacerbate and complicate preexisting respiratory diseases, like in the case of William.

The rapid degeneration of the American diet has led, in turn, to obesity, diabetes, allergy, asthma, sleep apnea, and reflux epidemics, all of which are essentially one and the same. It is long past time for physicians to address this problem.

In order to know if poor diet may be a factor or cause for a patient's symptoms, assess the patient's eating and drinking habits as a part of your history intake. As you ask questions about what your patients are habitually eating and drinking, counsel them and their parents to develop healthier dietary habits and decrease sugar intake.

We recommend you use the quizzes "How Do I Know My Child Has Reflux?" and the "Bad Reflux Diet," found on pages 12–13. Please feel free to adopt these quizzes as part of your practice. Have the patient's parents or other caregivers fill out the quizzes as part of the intake of new patients and upon each return visit. As the result of dietary modifications made based on the quiz results, we believe you will observe symptom reduction and treatment successes.

As we turn to the next parts of this book, chock full of helpful information and delicious recipes, we hope to have provided you, too, with information that will allow you to better identify and manage respiratory reflux in your patients.

Drs. Jamie Koufman, Julie Wei, and Karen Zur

PART I

UNDERSTANDING
REFLUX IN CHILDREN

CHAPTER 1

Acid Reflux: The Link Between Diet and Disease

When Dr. Jamie was a child in the 1950s, her mother put dinner on the table promptly at 6:00 p.m. like clockwork. Almost everything she prepared was locally grown. There were no soda machines or fast food restaurants, and rarely were acids and harmful chemicals used in foods and beverages as preservatives. Extra sugar wasn't added to anything except perhaps a cup of coffee. Almost for certain, young Dr. Jamie's diet—and the diets of many other families back then—was healthier than your family's diet is today.

Obesity, diabetes, heart disease, asthma, sleep apnea, osteoporosis, reflux, and esophageal cancer are all epidemics and major public health problems related to an unhealthy American diet. Reflux has increased 400 percent since 1975.[2] In the past two generations the arc of all of the above diseases has paralleled massive increases in the consumption of sugar, acids, and trans-fats, with the main culprits being soft drinks, snack foods and fast food.[4,5,10-18]

This book was written to help you understand some symptoms that otherwise healthy children may face and to set a blueprint to help you reclaim your child's health by changing the way you think about food. Reflux in children should be an essential focus for both doctors and the public in order to save millions of children from unnecessary medications and procedures. Reflux should be a focal point because it is fixable.

Dietary Acid Is a Problem

In 1973, in response to a serious outbreak of botulism, a potentially deadly type of food poisoning, Congress enacted the Low-Acid Canned Food Regulations Title 21 (21 CFR Part 113).[1,2] Under these regulations, the Food and Drug Administration (FDA) mandated that anything crossing state lines in a bottle or can must be acidic. From then on, acid was added to almost everything contained in a bottle or can in order to kill bacteria. In 1979, the FDA revised their recommendations and mandated that acidic canned food had to be at pH 4.6 or lower (21 CFR Part 114).[1]

Why a Low-Acid (Alkaline) Diet
Is Important for Refluxers

Throughout this book we will be recommending a low-acid diet as a strategy for fighting reflux. In truth, the single largest source of acid in our diet is from beverages in bottles and cans; nothing else we consume is as acidic, with the exception of lemons (pH 2.9) and limes (pH 2.7).[1]

When talking about the acidity of the food and drinks we consume, we refer to the pH scale. pH is a measure of how acidic or alkaline (aka basic, "basic" being the opposite of acidic) a liquid is. pH can be measured using a special instrument called a pH probe or with a pH strip, which is calibrated to reveal the exact pH of a substance. (For measurements in this book, we used an Apera Instruments SX610 waterproof pH pen tester.)

Acids and alkalines (bases) also have certain properties that make them more easily recognizable. Acids, vinegar (acetic acid) for example, are typically sour in taste, caustic, and elicit a burning sensation when smelled. Bases, like the ammonia contained in common household cleaners, are frequently bitter in taste, slippery to the touch, and reactive with grease and fats (think of how dish soap is helpful when cleaning a dirty pan).

How the pH (Acidity) Scale Works

The pH scale, used to measure acidity, is somewhat counterintuitive. pH 7 is neutral, meaning that the liquid is neither acidic nor alkaline. Anything below pH 7 is acidic; thus, the lower the number, the more acidic. Anything above pH 7 is alkaline; the higher the number, the more alkaline. pH 1 is very acidic, and caustics like bleach have values from pH 8 to14. Distilled water and most tap water is pH 7 (neutral), but vinegar, at pH 2.9, and lemon juice, at pH 2.7, are very acidic. For reference, the pH of stomach acid is pH 1 to 4. Also note that the pH scale is a logarithmic scale, like the Richter scale for measuring earthquakes, so that one point of difference actually represents an order of change ten-times stronger or weaker. For example, pH 4 is ten times more acidic than pH 5, and pH 4.8 is twice as acidic as 5.0. For this reason, simply diluting acidic beverages does not make them non-acidic.

Acids are added to foods and beverages in the form of ascorbic acid (a fancy term for vitamin C), citric acid, and phosphoric acid. (There are over fifty acids approved by the FDA as food additives; however, these three are the most common.[1]) Most fruit juices, already naturally acidic, have additional acid added to further lower the pH. When you see labels that read "all organic, all natural," they do not mean that no acid has been added. In fact, these labels may read, "Vitamin C Enhanced," indicating that ascorbic acid was added to further lower the pH.

Unfortunately, the FDA never told beverage manufacturers that too much acid might be harmful to consume. Today, the pH for most carbonated beverages ranges from 2.6 to 3.6, 10 to 100 times more acidic than required by law.[1,4] Have you ever heard of a soft drink beverage recall because of bacterial contamination? You haven't, because that level of acidity is strong enough to kill virtually everything. If you drink soda, you may be interested to know that the phosphoric acid some contain is also used in commercial rust remover.

Why Allow Children to Have This Inside Their Bodies?

A man claimed to have found a dead mouse in a bottle of Mountain Dew and sued the company. The defense of the soda manufacturer? That's impossible; you cannot find a dead mouse in Mountain Dew because the whole mouse would dissolve, bones, teeth, and all.[19]

Acid, Pepsin, and All That Jazz

For thirty years, Dr. Jamie's medical research has focused on the problem of reflux, unearthing many breakthrough discoveries.[1-4,20-68] When most people think about acid reflux, they envision stomach acid as the root cause of the disorder. That is only half true. The stuff that comes up out of the stomach, known as the refluxate, contains both acid and a nasty, destructive enzyme called pepsin.[1,4,24,42,44,54,58-62] Believe it or not, stomach acid isn't the main problem. In a way, the term "acid reflux" is misleading, since it is the digestive enzyme, pepsin, not acid, that causes most of the trouble.

This confusion occurs because pepsin can only do its job when acid is around to activate it. In an acidic environment, pepsin quickly and efficiently gets busy breaking down proteins into smaller, more easily digestible particles. Without acid to supercharge it, pepsin just isn't able to do its thing. On the other hand, acid-activated pepsin causes swelling and inflammation in human tissue, which in turn, lead to disease.

Here's the catch: Pepsin doesn't go away after you finish digesting your meal. It hangs around, and all it needs is some acid to wake it up again. While your stomach only produces acid when you eat a meal, pepsin doesn't care where the acid comes from—any acid will do.

Any foods you eat that are high in acid are perfectly sufficient for activating pepsin, and if there's no protein around that needs digesting, the pepsin will gnaw on whatever is handy—including the linings of your nose, throat and esophagus.[1-4,44,54,60,61] The saying, "You are what you eat" can be stated another way: "Be careful what you eat, because what you eat could be eating you!"

Imagine that your stomach is full of seawater and lobsters. The seawater is acid, and the lobsters (big, aggressive ones with mighty claws) are the pepsin molecules. When you reflux, the seawater splashes around. Some of it splashes upward into your throat. The lobsters ride this wave of seawater and attach themselves to the shore wherever they land—the shore being the delicate tissue and membranes lining your nose, throat, larynx (voice box), esophagus, and lungs.

The lobsters are hanging on by their claws. It doesn't really matter now whether the seawater they need for survival splashes up from below or pours down from above. To these lobsters, it's all just a rejuvenating splash. Once a pepsin molecule is bound to, say, your throat, any dietary source of acid—soda pop, salsa, strawberries—can reactivate it.

Many doctors mistakenly believe that pepsin is only active below pH 4. Nothing could be further from the truth. Pepsin does maximum damage at pH 2 (100 percent activity), but it can still do significant damage in an environment of up to pH 5.[54,62]

When pepsin binds to tissue, it remains stable for a long time.[54] The question is not whether it is active, but how active. All those popular and expensive anti-reflux medicines don't actually turn off the acid, they just turn it down, reduce it somewhat. On television, you'll see those little acid pumps in the stomach give up at the sight of a powerful purple pill, but that's not what really happens.

Despite the strongest anti-reflux medications, known as proton pump inhibitors (PPIs, e.g., Prilosec, Protonix, Nexium, Dexilant, omeprazole, lansoprazole, esomeprazole), the stomach will continue to churn out a significant amount of acid. More than 50 percent of people with respiratory reflux who try PPIs do not respond to them,[41,69] and another 10 to 15 percent get side effects including nausea, gas, bloating, diarrhea, and abdominal pain. We still don't have a universally effective anti-reflux medication. The best medications we have are only mediocre acid-suppressants, and they don't eradicate pepsin. Until now, what has been missing from the treatment equation is an understanding of the profound impact of dietary acid. To correct this misunderstanding, what follows is a scientific summary of exactly how reflux causes problems:

- Acid and pepsin work together to cause reflux-related symptoms and diseases.

- None of the available anti-reflux medications turns off acid completely.

- When pepsin attaches to human tissue, inflammation and disease may result.

- Dietary acid can activate pepsin that is already present in or on tissue.

- Tissues injured by reflux need a period of recovery, requiring a low-acid, alkaline diet.

It is important to re-emphasize that most children with reflux have silent respiratory reflux that is often not easily detected. Acid reflux is not simply limited to heartburn and indigestion, and when it masquerades as something else, everyone, including doctors, gets confused.

The entire rationale of an alkaline diet is to suffocate and kill the lobsters (pepsin molecules) lingering in the nose, throat, and lungs by avoiding acidic food items such as fruit juice, soda, and citrus. Throughout this book, we recommend a detailed plan to adjust your children's dietary and eating habits at every stage of their development.

A normal pH in the throats of healthy children (and adults) is around 6.8; however, in children who have respiratory reflux, it can be up to 100 times more acidic, down to a pH of around 4.8. This can lead to injury to throat tissue, and really, tissues anywhere in the respiratory tract. The membranes lining the respiratory tract, called "mucous membranes," respond to inflammation by getting swollen and producing more mucus. This swelling and inflammation, in addition to the actual tissue damage caused by reflux, can lead to all of the many symptoms and conditions listed on page 12.

When initially transitioning to a low-acid diet, you may want to try to have your children eat and drink only foods and beverages that are above a pH of 5.0.[1-4] Try this for two weeks. You can apply this system to baby food as well. We realize this is not easy. Try your best. For babies, we have provided a list of the pH of different baby foods as well as fresh fruits and vegetables on pages 34–36. Try to create your own shopping list for some less acidic choices. In general, just remember, the less acidic and higher the pH, the better.

pH Balancing

Remember, those lobsters (pepsin molecules) thrive in acid. For this reason, if something acidic is consumed, it should be "chased" by something alkaline. The idea of pH balancing is to combine acidic foods with alkaline foods to reduce the overall acidity of a meal. For example, putting somewhat acidic fruit like strawberries in breakfast cereal with milk (e.g. cow, almond, soy) or in oatmeal achieves pH balance, because all types of milk and oatmeal are alkaline. Acid and alkaline cancel each other out, which equates to pH balancing.

Alkaline water, with its unique health benefits for children and adults suffering from reflux, is one amazing product that is rapidly gaining in popularity. Natural alkaline water comes from underground sources, with a pH as high as 8 to 11 (due to the presence of limestone and calcium carbonate). No other food or beverage found in nature is as alkaline, making it a fantastic tool for neutralizing acid and combating reflux by achieving pH balance.

In laboratory experiments, it has been shown that the pepsin molecule breaks down at a pH of 8 or higher.[65] For this reason, drinking alkaline water is particularly good for reflux, because it not only neutralizes the "sea water," it kills the "lobsters," washing them out of the tissues of the throat and esophagus.

We recommend drinking alkaline water as a partial treatment for both children and adults with reflux. Alkaline water is the ultimate pH-balancing beverage and is completely safe in every way. There are no downsides to drinking alkaline water. To find it, look in your local grocery store for one that is pH 8 or higher. The pH is usually shown on the label. You might have to go to a specialty grocery store, or you can always order an alkaline water pitcher online as an alternative. Check out cerrawater.com.

How Reflux Develops

First and foremost, our bodies (stomachs) naturally make acid, and we consume foods that either naturally contain acid or are purposely acidified for preservation purposes. In order to better understand what is happening when we discuss acid reflux, let's take a basic look at how we normally swallow and digest our food.

Normal physiology of the swallowing process starts in the mouth where, after food is chewed and formed into a bolus (ball), at the initiation of the swallow, it is pushed by the tongue to the back of the upper throat (pharynx). Infants on a liquid diet use the same mechanism to push liquid down the throat. Next, the tongue and pharyngeal muscles contract like a piston, gently driving the bolus further down, toward the upper end of the food pipe (esophagus), located just behind the voice box (larynx).

At the beginning of the swallow, the back of the nose (nasopharynx) and the trap-door-like cartilage above the voice box (epiglottis) close, so that liquid or food do not go back up into the nose (yuck) or accidentally into the voice box (larynx) and then down the windpipe (trachea). Our swallowing is designed to go one place: into the esophagus. If food somehow enters the windpipe (aspiration), coughing occurs as your body's means of dislodging the irritant. If it fails to do so, pneumonia may result. (For more on aspiration, see pages 186–187.) Normally, once the food or liquid makes it to the bottom of the throat where it joins the esophagus, a valve called the upper esophageal sphincter (UES) relaxes so that the bolus can enter the esophagus. Once the bolus is in the esophagus, the entire muscular esophageal tube contracts to push the bolus downward toward the stomach. Picture a cobra that just swallowed an egg.

At the bottom of the esophagus is another valve, the lower esophageal sphincter (LES) The job of the LES is to open, allowing the bolus to enter the stomach, closing tightly after it passes to keep food and liquid from coming back up into the esophagus, from refluxing.

Reflux occurs when the LES inappropriately re-opens after eating or drinking. When reflux travels all the way up above the UES, into the throat, we call that respiratory reflux or laryngopharyngeal reflux (LPR). (LPR literally means "backflow into the voice-box and throat" from the stomach.) As previously mentioned, the new and better term for LPR is "respiratory reflux." (Today, the terms respiratory reflux and LPR are used interchangeably.)

Respiratory reflux is the diagnosis we most often consider when treating children who present with acid reflux aliases such as noisy breathing, recurrent croup, "asthma," chronic nose stuffiness or runniness, and "allergies." By the way, not all reflux is acidic. We may also regurgitate non-acidic food from the stomach that can sometimes be as irritating to the body as acid reflux. Once in the stomach, our children's foods and beverages should stay there.

Reflux may occur when the LES is too loose, either not squeezing tightly enough or relaxing too often when it should not. There are many foods and medications that have the side effect of relaxing the LES. Foods and beverages that are high in acid, caffeine, peppermint, citrus, chocolate, sugar, and fat have been shown to make the LES relax. The looser the LES, the more our one-way digestive tract becomes two-way. For newborns, the LES is sometimes underdeveloped, making it loose in the first place, which we will discuss in Chapter 3.

Childhood Obesity and Reflux

Here are some shocking facts about childhood obesity, according to the Center for Disease Control (2017) and others.[70-75]

- Obesity affects about 12.7 million children and adolescents in the United States.
- Childhood obesity has more than doubled in children and tripled in adolescents in the past three decades.
- As of 2016, about 20 percent of children and adolescents (ages 6–19) were overweight or obese.
- Obesity in childhood is associated with subsequent obesity in adults, chronic medical diseases, and higher medical costs.[75-77]

We know childhood obesity is an epidemic, but what isn't as widely understood is its linkage to reflux. A 2006 study reported that the risk of reflux is directly related to body mass index (BMI), the standard measure of obesity.[75] This report suggested that moderate amounts of weight gain may result in the development of reflux. This is, of course, concerning in light of the overall rise of obesity in the United States.

In another recent study looking at the correlation between reflux and obesity in children, researchers found that reflux was highly associated with obesity; that is, obese children are more likely to have respiratory reflux than lean children.[77] Obese children had a higher incidence of "asthma," but what was found when testing them for "asthma" was that they did not actually have it.[75] What these children did have was respiratory reflux that had been falsely attributed to "asthma." Imagine all of the medicines that these kids were on to treat a disease they didn't even have. This is important on so many levels, from possible side effects, to the cost of unneeded medicines, loss of time from school, and continued suffering.

The American Association of Pediatrics (AAP) has provided practical recommendations for obesity prevention including changing the food parents bring into the home, reducing sedentary behaviors, avoiding screen time, and identifying opportunities for increasing activity to sixty minutes a day.[77]

Judging by the results of these studies, if the rate of obesity could be reduced, then the rates of reflux and reflux-related symptoms such as "asthma" could be diminished—food for thought!

How Do I Know If My Child Has Reflux?

Many of your child's symptoms and respiratory illnesses may actually be due to acid reflux. Even serious medical problems that require physician care can be reflux-caused.

Take the two quizzes on the following pages to see if your child has reflux.

Disclaimer: The quizzes on the next two pages do not provide a medical diagnosis; they are intended to simply help parents consider the possibility of acid reflux as a problem.

Does My Child Have Acid Reflux?
The Pediatrics Reflux Index©

Circle all that apply to your child's symptoms or current diagnosis on a scale of 0 to 5. (0, if not at all; 5, being severe).

Asthma	0	1	2	3	4	5
Stuffy nose	0	1	2	3	4	5
Runny nose	0	1	2	3	4	5
Ear infections	0	1	2	3	4	5
Sinus infections	0	1	2	3	4	5
Nasal congestion	0	1	2	3	4	5
Recurrent croup	0	1	2	3	4	5
Noisy breathing	0	1	2	3	4	5
Chronic cough	0	1	2	3	4	5
Spitting up	0	1	2	3	4	5
Always has a "cold"	0	1	2	3	4	5
Raspy voice	0	1	2	3	4	5
Obesity	0	1	2	3	4	5

Total _____

Add up the circled numbers at the bottom to get your child's Pediatrics Reflux Index. If the total PRI score is more than 10, chances are your child has reflux

Notes & Recommendations

_____

_____

_____

_____

_____

Your Child's Unhealthy "Bad Reflux Diet" Quiz©

Circle all that apply (scale is 0 to 5 servings/glasses per day; if more than five, write in the number on the line provided.)

Milk/flavored milk	0	1	2	3	4	5 ____
Sweet tea	0	1	2	3	4	5 ____
Soda	0	1	2	3	4	5 ____
Sports drinks	0	1	2	3	4	5 ____
Energy drinks	0	1	2	3	4	5 ____
Fruit juice	0	1	2	3	4	5 ____
Fruit punch	0	1	2	3	4	5 ____
Lemonade	0	1	2	3	4	5 ____
Pouched drinks	0	1	2	3	4	5 ____
Ice cream	0	1	2	3	4	5 ____
Candy	0	1	2	3	4	5 ____
Cookies	0	1	2	3	4	5 ____
Yogurt	0	1	2	3	4	5 ____

Total _____

Add up the circled numbers to get your child's Bad Reflux Diet Score; a score of 10 or more suggests that your child has a "high-risk" Bad Reflux Diet.

Notes & Recommendations

_____

_____

_____

_____

_____

CHAPTER 2

Reflux Simplified:
A Kid-Friendly Conversation

The information in the previous chapter may be too complex to share with most children. What follows is a composite conversation between Dr. Jamie and her grandchildren about digestion, nutrition, and acid reflux, a conversation we recommend you initiate with your children. This chapter is intended as a resource to help parents communicate these concepts: Read it to your child out loud (when s/he is old enough to understand), or explain it in your own words. (The children's responses are depicted in "quotations" below.)

Do you know what makes you grow bigger, stronger, and taller? It's food. Food is the fuel your body needs to build strong muscles and bones and all the other parts of your body.

When you eat food, it goes through a process called *digestion*, which is how the body turns the food we eat into the fuel your body needs. There are three types of fuel that you get from food: protein, sugar, and fat. You also get vitamins and minerals from food, too.

Vitamins and minerals help your body grow and stay healthy just as much as protein, sugar, and fat. You need all five of those things to grow up big and strong. Those are the parts that make up your *nutrition*. So, when you eat food, your body takes in those five good parts. Do you remember them?

"Yes, protein, sugar, and fat."

And don't forget vitamins and minerals. Vitamins and minerals help build strong bones and make sure all of our organ systems, like our hearts, lungs, and brains, work correctly. Vitamins and minerals are like helpers for the protein, sugar, and fat you get from food. What about the food that your body doesn't use? Do you know what happens to the rest?

"It's poop, right?"

Yes. The body takes out the good parts of food, and the rest becomes poop.

Do you remember the five parts of nutrition, still?

"Yup! Vitamins, minerals, fat, sugar and protein."

Very good! And remember all five are part of the nutrition you need to stay healthy and grow. You can think of nutrition as the "good stuff" you get from food.

I want to talk more about *digestion*. Digestion is the way your body gets nutrition. For you to get your nutrition, you first have to digest your food. Here's how digestion works: After you take a bite of food and chew it up, you swallow, and your tongue and throat push the food into the swallowing tube (called the esophagus) that connects your throat with your stomach.

As food travels downwards, a trap door (called a valve) opens to let it pass through, into the stomach. After the food gets in, the trap door usually closes so that the food stays in the stomach and cannot go back up the swallowing tube.

The stomach makes strong acid to help mush up (partially digest) the food. (This strong acid in the stomach is important, as you will see in a minute.) Finally, the stomach pushes the food into your intestines, which look like a long hose that's neatly packed inside your belly.

The intestines are where the fuel we have talked about (nutrition) enters and is taken up by your body. The intestines are like strainers that allow the five parts of nutrition—vitamins, minerals, fat, sugar, and protein—to enter the rest of your body, while keeping the leftover odds and ends out. And the parts of the food you don't use, remember what happens to that?

(Giggling) "POOP!"

Right! It is in the intestines where the digested food enters your body. Guess how long your intestines are?

"1,000 feet?"

No, not that long. They're about twenty-two feet long. That's longer than this room!

Remember, nutrition is your body's energy and fuel. Food is what makes you grow bigger, stronger, and taller each year, and digestion is how your body takes the food and turns it into fuel. So, before we go on, can you tell me what you've learned about *digestion* and *nutrition*?

"When we eat food, our stomachs mush it up with acid, and it goes into our long intestines . . . we get our nutrition . . . in our intestines . . . the good part of our food . . . vitamins, minerals, protein, fat, and sugar . . . then, we poop!"

Wow, that was great! Now that you understand nutrition and digestion, let's start talking about *acid reflux*. Remember the trap door between the esophagus and the stomach? When that trap door opens up and allows acid and mushed-up food to escape your stomach and travel the wrong way, up into your throat and mouth, that's *acid reflux*. The word *reflux* actually means "back-flow." Do you remember when the toilet backed up and water got all over the floor? That was a sort of reflux.

Acid reflux is all about the stomach, the acid, and the trap door between the stomach and the swallowing tube. If that trap door opens when the stomach is still full of acid and mushed-up food that then comes back up the swallowing tube, we call that *acid reflux*.

This can happen especially at night, when you lie down to go to sleep. That's when all the stuff in the stomach, acid and all, comes up into your throat. It is especially bad if you ate just before bed, because the food hasn't had a chance to be digested and will come back up, along with the acid. Can you imagine what happens when you have acid reflux?

"I would throw up?"

That's right, but you might not know that you're throwing up if you are asleep. You might, instead, wake up having trouble breathing, if the vomit went into your throat or lungs. There are lots of other bad things that acid might do to your body. The next day, you might have problems breathing out of a stuffy or runny nose.

Acid reflux can also cause you to get ear infections, fits of coughing, and have trouble swallowing, too. It might feel like you throw up inside your throat and then swallow it back down. Have you ever felt this happen? Let's take a quick and easy quiz together now, to see if you have any of the problems that acid reflux can cause. Let's check off the symptoms that apply to you.

- Asthma
- Hard time breathing
- Trouble breathing when exercising
- Stuffy nose
- Tonsillitis
- Runny nose
- Ear infections

- Sinus infections
- Too much mucus/phlegm
- Nasal congestion
- Noisy breathing
- Chronic cough
- Always have a "cold"
- Raspy voice
- Being overweight

You know, not everyone knows about acid reflux like we do. Not everybody, meaning not every parent; not even every doctor knows as much about acid reflux as you do now. Now that you know what to look out for, if you have acid reflux, what should you do?

It's easy: Acid reflux can be corrected simply by eating healthier food and changing the time when you eat. Remember that trap door between the swallowing tube and the stomach? Unhealthy food makes that valve go to sleep on the job and allows whatever is in your stomach to travel backwards, up into your swallowing tube. What unhealthy foods do you enjoy that might lead to acid reflux? Let's take the food quiz (on page 13) and see how you do, okay?

There are many foods and sugary drinks that taste so good when you eat them, but are not healthy and have too much sugar and fat in them. That's why they're so delicious! As a rule, sugar and fats as in packaged cookies and chips increase acid reflux.

The fruits, vegetables, and foods we cook in the kitchen are less likely to cause reflux. On the next page there are five things that we can do together to help decrease acid reflux, so that you can grow stronger and healthier and avoid needing to go to the doctor (and even yucky medicines!).

Here are "Five Fabulous Tips" for Healthy Eating

1. You are probably not going to like this one: No bedtime snacks. Let's stop eating and drinking (water is okay) for at least one-and-a-half hours before your bedtime. Make sure to use the bathroom before you go to sleep.

2. You cannot drink juice or any other sugary drink more than once a day, and soda pop almost never or only on special occasions. Pouched drinks and sweet tea are out too. Anything that's not water has lots of sugar in it. Also, not too much milk (especially strawberry or chocolate milk) because it causes reflux. It is best to drink water, most of the time, every day. Water is the best thing you can drink. Do you like drinking water?

3. We are going to cut down on eating fast food and eat a lot fewer hot dogs, hamburgers, pizza, tomato sauce, garlicy/oniony food, and lunchmeats.

4. You can have sweets or junk food just once a day. That includes cookies, ice cream, chips, cheese, and sweet breakfast cereals.

5. Everyone should eat 4 to 5 servings a day of fruits and vegetables. Red apples, pears, melons, grapes, figs, dates, and bananas are all tasty snacks, and the healthiest veggies are broccoli, green beans, asparagus, Brussels sprouts, and of course, salads.

We as a family are going to try to eat in a healthier way. When we can, I want to take you with me to the grocery store, and I would *love* to have you help me cook dinner.

Does all this make sense? Do you understand reflux now?

"Yes, I get it!"

CHAPTER 3

Newborn to Age Two

For brand-new and veteran parents alike, being spit on, peed on, and, yes, even pooped on is an accepted and expected parental rite of passage. From burp clothes to BPA-free (biphenol-A-free plastic) products, to the sizes, shapes, and flow-speeds of bottle nipples, parents are consumed by what to put into their babies' bodies—and how it comes out!

For at least the first two years of your child's life, you will watch like a hawk how well s/he sleeps, eats, naps, and poops. When asked the common question, "Is she a good baby?" (as if there could ever be such a thing as a bad one) your likely response will rely on two factors: how well s/he eats, and how well s/he sleeps. Most of the time, these two functions are intertwined. The more comfortable your baby's body feels, the better s/he sleeps.

In this section, we aim to answer the most common questions we hear as pediatric ear, nose, and throat specialists about baby nutrition and feeding and to offer new insights on what may be the insidious root of your baby's woes, something so basic that it is usually overlooked and taken for granted, especially in children ages newborn to two years—acid reflux.

Acid Reflux Isn't Just for Old Men and Pregnant Ladies

Dr. Harvey Karp, author of the bestselling book series, *The Happiest Baby*, made famous the concept of the fourth trimester. "Our babies aren't like horses. They can't run the first day of life," Karp says. "And so, we need to recognize that they're evicted from the womb three months before they're ready for the world."[78]

Dr. Karp is exactly right! Newborn brains are not fully developed, nor are their lungs, skeletal system, teeth, eyesight, or digestive tracts. In fact, it's hard to believe that with all of their limitations, babies are able to coordinate breathing and eating functions as well as they do. With all that growing still ahead, there are bound to be a few glitches. As a parent, it's a matter of recognizing what's normal and what isn't.

As mentioned earlier, at the bottom of the esophagus, where it connects to the stomach, there is a valve called the lower esophageal sphincter

(LES). One explanation of why reflux occurs is that the LES can be too loose, either not squeezing tightly enough or relaxing too often when it shouldn't. There are many reasons for this to occur. One of them is that newborns and infants, especially those who are born too early or prematurely, may need more time for the LES to grow stronger.

This fact does not diminish the seriousness of the underlying problem. Reflux can affect the wellbeing of some babies and children to the point where some need to see doctors for medical treatment, to make sure they remain healthy and growing. Terms such as "spitting up," "posseting," "regurgitation," and "spilling" are all descriptions of reflux. Spitting up, which occurs daily in about fifty percent of infants younger than three months of age, usually subsides without medical treatment in healthy infants by twelve to fourteen months of age.[79-83]

Normal Versus Pathological (Abnormal) Reflux

So, how much spitting up is normal? Described as "physiological," normal reflux occurs when a living organism or its bodily parts function as expected. When reflux is described as pathological (pathos meaning sad or pitiful), this is not the case.

Physiologically, as infants nurse or drink either breast milk or formula from a bottle, with each swallow, they also swallow some air. For this very reason you have probably stood paralyzed when trying to make heads or tails out of the plethora of bottle and nipple choices promising your child reduced air intake.

When air is swallowed, gas bubbles build up during feeding, which is why we burp our children. Spit up occurs when gas bubbles force up some breast milk or formula during burping. Again, some spitting up after feeding is normal, and many times you'll notice it doesn't seem to bother your baby. It can even sometimes come out of your baby's nose, and that can be normal, too, albeit, not pretty. There isn't a hard line between normal and abnormal spit up, and the difference between spitting up and vomiting is determined by the amount of the spit up and when it occurs. Some spitting up after feeding and even occasional vomiting, particularly after a big feed, is physiological (normal).

Frequent vomiting associated with breathing problems like stuffy nose or noisy breathing, vomiting during the night, and projectile vomiting are usually considered pathological or abnormal. When a baby has trouble breathing, s/he works harder to suck in air, and, as a side effect, stomach content may be siphoned off of the esophagus, back into the throat, causing the baby to vomit. Another source of pathological reflux is if there is a problem with the digestive tract itself, such as a twisting of the stomach or a narrowing of the valve that allows the stomach to empty into the small intestine. The latter condition is called pyloric stenosis (page 190). Newborn babies who have projectile vomiting after every feeding should be evaluated by a physician for this problem, since it requires surgery, but is ultimately fixable. Your doctor might have asked you if you or your partner had pyloric stenosis when you were born, as it tends to run in families. Projectile vomiting requires medical attention. If this happens to your baby, see your pediatrician *pronto*.

Both physiological and pathological reflux can be jarring, especially for unseasoned parents. What makes it worse is the inability of the child to describe to you how s/he is feeling, which is why we refer to children as "silent refluxers." As a new parent, you quickly become an expert in reading body language. When babies cry, we tend to think that they are either wet or hungry, and usually try to offer a feeding.

There are signs to help determine whether your baby is hungry or in pain. If your child stiffens his body like a board, arches his back, puts his head to the side, has a swollen/distended belly, winces, or flails his legs or arms, consider it a signal that something is abnormal and talk to your pediatrician.

In toddler-age children, signs of pain might be pulling their hair or ears or rubbing their face. Be aware that sometimes symptoms of acid reflux are subtle or disguised by a completely different, seemingly unrelated problem or alias.

The Many Aliases of Acid Reflux in Infants

Runny Nose & Nasal Congestion

One of the most common concerns of parents of infants is nasal congestion and stuffiness. Babies are small, and that means everything is smaller, including all of their breathing passages (nasal passages, mouth, and throat areas), so they are more susceptible to congestion. Infant noses are so small that even the slightest mucus buildup or swelling can be a nuisance. Some parents simply can't seem to stop gooey boogers from streaming out of their child's nostrils, and with bad blowing skills continuing through toddlerdom, mucus and stuffiness become ever more frequent.

Since an infant's anatomy is small, with little distance between the head and the stomach, reflux doesn't have to go very far, which is why reflux of breast milk or formula can so easily come up into the nose. This can cause irritation, excess mucus production, and swelling inside the nose. If excess mucus dries up to become crusty boogers that clog up their baby's little nostrils, parents will hear this congestion as strange breathing noises, even whistling.

Babies Are Obligate Nose Breathers

Did you know that babies have to breathe through their noses for the first four months of life? That's what being an obligate nasal breather means; infants literally need to breathe in that manner. The lack of ability to compensate by breathing through the mouth is why nasal congestion can pose a serious breathing problem for infants.

One mother described her son as having a phlegmy "smoker's cough," and was shocked when we told her that her baby didn't have a cold or a bronchial problem but acid reflux. The congested sounds that reflux babies make as they breathe can also go hand in hand with a thick nasal discharge that, no matter how hard you try, can't be cleared out with a suction bulb.

Allergies

Parents of babies with chronically stuffy noses tend to see physicians wondering if their child has allergies. We see many children less than two years of age with nasal symptoms that are attributed to "allergies," but despite allergy medications, their symptoms stubbornly persist. In actuality, the development of environmental allergies to allergens such as trees, grasses, pollen, dust mites, and mold takes many years. Parents often believe that the underlying problem is "allergy," simply because their pediatrician mistakenly put their baby on an allergy medication in the first place.

Some babies do develop allergies to caseins, which are proteins found in cow's milk. Even when not allergic, many babies (and adults, for that matter) have sensitivity to it. Often, people think it is lactose in milk that they are not tolerating, when, in most cases, it is the casein that is the culprit. Note that in addition to nasal congestion, reactions to cow's milk may

Bowel Movements and Constipation

According to the American Academy of Pediatrics (AAP), most children have one to two bowl movements each day, but others may have only one every three days. As long as a child appears comfortable passing the stools and is not in pain, having a bowel movement every three days may be normal for them. Breastfed babies usually have mustard-looking watery poop. Formula-fed babies have a pastier stool, usually earth-toned colors from yellow to green to brown.[85] In babies who are over one month old and non-breastfed, constipation is considered when there is no bowel movement in three or more days, or if there is significant straining to get the stool out. In a constipated baby, the stool may look like pellets. This may be a sign of sensitivity to newly introduced food, milk products, or an ingredient in the formula. If your baby has multiple diapers with pellets of stool, or if the stool has blood in it, let your pediatrician know. It is also recommended that you contact your pediatrician if your child's stool is white or red. The AAP has online resources via healthychildren.org to help monitor your baby's stooling habits as well as guidelines of when to contact your pediatrician.[85]

include bloody stools, constipation, diarrhea, bloating, and other gastrointestinal symptoms.

Infants and toddlers with chronic nasal symptoms are often given too much milk, juice, and sugary beverages, while many may have inappropriate bedtime snacks such as milk and cookies. Their "allergies" are among the most common misdiagnoses in the children who see us for second or third opinions. Reflux induced by unhealthy beverages is often the only correct diagnosis.

If your infant or toddler is always congested and full of snot, think respiratory reflux, and closely examine your baby's diet for acidic or other reflux-causing foods and beverages (see pages 13).

Noisy Breathing

Remember, infants are obligate nose breathers until about four months of age. For this reason, nasal congestion can result in noisy breathing as a baby struggles to take in air. It is usually pretty easy to tell if a snotty nose is the problem. If your infant has nasal congestion, s/he may have trouble breathing. While this demands a visit to the pediatrician, be on alert for an incorrect diagnosis of asthma, and consider that acid reflux, often under-diagnosed, is the most likely cause.

Other breathing conditions are important to consider. Croup is usually associated with a cold, a viral infection that causes swelling of the voice box, windpipe, and even the lungs. This swelling narrows the air passages, and as air is being pushed out against semi-closed vocal cords, suddenly the voice box opens, creating a "barking" or "croupy" cough. When the infection is severe, children sometimes need to be hospitalized. Viral croup can be very scary in young children. If there is any question about the severity of any breathing problem, take your child to your pediatrician or an emergency room right away.

Some children have recurrent croup, frequently awakening from sleep with a croupy cough. This may happen several times a year or even several times a week. This type of croup is usually caused by acid reflux into the voice box. Recurrent nighttime croup without a fever? Think reflux.

Finally, there are both congenital and acquired conditions that can narrow an infant's breathing passages anywhere from the upper throat to the lungs. These problems present either right after birth (up to four weeks) or worsen progressively over time. True medical emergencies may result from structural narrowing of the airway (see pages 175–187). If your child's breathing gets worse over time, even with adjustments in feedings, s/he may have a growth or scarring in the respiratory tract. Talk to your pediatrician; you may need to see a pediatric otolaryngologist to have the airway examined.

If something does not seem right, get your pediatrician involved in the conversation, have your baby evaluated, and come up with a plan. Here are some serious symptoms and signs to look out for:

- Abnormal bowl movements
- Choking during meals
- Fevers with wheezing
- Not gaining weight or losing weight
- Pauses in breathing while asleep (sleep apnea)
- Persistent coughing
- Projectile vomiting
- Recurrent pneumonias

- Significant eczema
- Swollen or tense stomach

With babies, your partnership with your pediatrician is important in order to ensure that your child is meeting the expected milestones for development, weight gain, and health. If along the way you feel that something isn't right, trust your intuition and reach out to your pediatrician.

Nursing, Formula, and Baby Food, Oh My! Are You Making Your Baby's Reflux Worse?

The emphases of this book are nutrition, diet, and lifestyle. When it comes to your infant's health, there are things you may or may not be doing that could exacerbate your baby's acid reflux. Here we turn to lifestyle issues and decisions new parents face, including breastfeeding, napping, formulas, baby food and sleeping habits. All are areas of your parenting life that are easy to assess and change if necessary.

Breastfeeding

If your parental instincts and your newfound body-language-interpreting skills tell you that your baby is not comfortable around feeding time, consider monitoring what you are eating and drinking. What mothers eat and drink is transferred to the baby through breast milk. Your baby can suffer from the same reflux as you. Most mothers end up looking for patterns and choosing to eliminate foods that correlate with how much spitting up and fussiness their baby seems to have.

You may find that pizza, spicy meals, dairy products, certain meats, and other types of foods that cause discomfort in your body, may be affecting your baby in much the same fashion. Most mothers will recall that during pregnancy, as their bellies got bigger, they experienced acid reflux from the pressure put on their stomach by the baby. Some also remember that certain foods and drinks seemed to cause extra reflux during this time.

Mothers who cannot produce enough milk but desire their baby to receive the benefits of breastfeeding may join a pool of donated milk in order to feed their baby. For this reason, the dietary information of the lactating mother may not be known. If you are in situation in which you think your baby is refluxing and suspect the possibility of breast milk sensitivity, consider using another donor, or if you know the donor, ask about her dietary habits.

Formula

Not every mother decides to take the route of breastfeeding. For generations, babies have been fed formula and have turned out just fine. Nevertheless, just like sensitivity to products transferred through a mother's breast milk can cause a baby to have reflux, so can formulas. When a baby comes to the specialist's office experiencing feeding difficulties, many possibilities come up. Does the baby have a tongue tie? Is she swallowing too much air? Have you tried the bottles with straws that can reduce the amount of air swallowed during feeds? Is the nose too stuffy for your baby to feed properly?

If none of these issues is identified, ask your doctor about switching to a different formula. It's possible your baby is sensitive to your current one. There are many different types of formulas and brands. Ask your doctor about a formula option that requires less digestion on your baby's part (hypoallergenic formulas), referred to as "protein hydrolysate formulas." These formulas contain milk protein that has been heated up to cause it to break (hydrolyze) into smaller protein products that are more easily digested. This option may be better for babies with cow's milk or soy allergies. Some formulas that are partially hydrolyzed include Alimentum (Similac) and Nutramigen (Enfamil).

In one study of formula-fed infants, reflux symptoms resolved in twenty-four percent of infants after a two-week trial of receiving a protein hydrolysate formula, thickened with one tablespoon rice cereal per ounce of formula, while avoiding overfeeding, seated and supine (laying on back) positions, and free of environmental tobacco smoke.[86] In very severe cases of protein allergies, some babies need to be fed amino-acid-based formulas. These are completely hydrolyzed formulas where the protein is fully broken down into its building block components, called amino acids, before consumption. Examples of this type of formula are: Neocate (Nutricia), EleCare (Abbott), and PurAmino (Enfamil).

With these tips in mind, you will hopefully find that spitting up and difficulties with feedings subside with less back arching, more regular bowel movements, and diminished fussiness. You should especially consider hypoallergenic formulas if your baby regurgitates and gets skin eczema. Eczema could be a marker of a sensitivity or allergy-type reaction to the milk or formula.[87]

If all else fails, talk to your pediatrician about the need for further evaluation or management of reflux. We try to avoid recommending reflux medications in young babies, but if a baby is having medical issues such as poor weight gain, breathing problems, laryngomalacia (noisy breathing from floppiness in the cartilages of the voice box), or aspiration (liquid going into the windpipe and lungs, which can cause infection/pneumonia) a visit to a specialist such as a pediatric otolaryngologist, gastroenterologist (GI), or pulmonologist may be in order.

It is uncommon though sometimes necessary for babies to need medicines or surgeries for their reflux. The two main categories of acid-reducing medications are H2-antagonists and proton pump inhibitors; a third option is prokinetic agents, medications that promote faster emptying of the stomach.

When prescribing medications for your baby, your doctor should share the duration of the proposed plan. Some medications can be ended abruptly, while others must be slowly weaned. As all medications have side effects, be sure to always ask your doctor which symptoms and signs you should watch for. Be sure to report side effects to your doctor when and if they occur.

For severe reflux problems, your doctor may refer you to a pediatric surgeon to discuss a surgical procedure to "tighten" your baby's LES. Usually, medical treatment is tried first to avoid this surgery. Be sure to discuss all options with your baby's pediatrician or specialists. The topic of anti-reflux medication and surgery is further addressed in Appendix A, page 171.

Baby Food

Have you ever tasted the baby food in jars that say "turkey and gravy" or "spaghetti and meatballs"? If you have, we are fairly certain you would not be feeding them to your baby. Consider how acidic, processed, and unnatural most baby foods in a jar have to be in order to not spoil[1] on a shelf without refrigeration for many months or years. Look at the expiration date! "Homemade" turkey and gravy simply doesn't last nearly that long. We suggest that you shouldn't be trusting of labels nor assume that processed food is safe and good for your baby.

Ascorbic acid ("vitamin C"), folic acid, and/or citric acid are often added to jar foods to help preserve them by decreasing the risk of bacteria growing in the product. The FDA mandates keeping the pH of jar food less than 4.6 so it does not spoil; however, some products have a much lower pH, making them even more acidic.[1] For a refresher on pH levels, see page 4. For now, just remember, the higher the pH, the better.

Acidity (pH) Testing Results of Common Formulas and Baby Foods

Dr. Karen went to local grocery stores and pharmacies and purchased all of the products tested (shown below). Obviously, she couldn't test every product available on the market.

The pH of these products was measured using the Apera Instruments SX610 Waterproof pH pen tester, which has a ±0.1 pH accuracy. Its range is 0 to 14.0 pH, and it has a replaceable probe. The pH meter was calibrated with a buffer solution of 7.0 pH and recalibrated as needed. In between measurements, the probe tip was gently rinsed in water and dried. When the pH reading was 7.0, the next product was tested.

The tables below were organized based on the pH reading of each item. The higher the pH reading, the better it is from a reflux and pepsin interaction standpoint. We recommend food that is pH 5 or more but will accept a pH as low as 4.5.

Formulas and Shakes (None of those below is acidic)

Brand	Description	pH
Pediasure	Grow & Gain: Strawberry Shake	7.0
Enfamil	Infant formula: Gentlease	6.8
Enfamil	Infant formula: Infant	6.8
Enfamil	Infant formula: Newborn–3 mos.	6.7
Similac	Sensitive	6.7
Similac	Infant formula with Iron Pro-Advance	6.4

Examples of Least Acidic Baby Foods

Brand	Description	pH
Gerber	Green Beans	5.9
Gerber	Squash	5.9
Beech Nut	Turkey Rice Dinner	5.7
Beech Nut	Mixed Vegetables	5.4
Earth's Best	Organic Garden Vegetables	5.4
Gerber	Chicken Noodle	5.3
Earth's Best	Organic Spinach & Potatoes	5.3
Beech Nut	Corn & Sweet Potatoes	5.3
Earth's Best	Organic Corn & Butternut Squash	5.3
Gerber	Sweet Potatoes	5.2

Examples of Most Acidic Baby Foods

Brand	Description	pH
Gerber	Applesauce	3.7
Gerber	Apple Blueberry	3.7
Earth's Best	Organic First Apples	3.8
Beech Nut	Applesauce	3.9
Beech Nut	Pears & Raspberries	3.9
Gerber	Pears	4.0
Gerber	Prunes	4.0
Gerber	Peaches	4.0
Beech Nut	Rice Cereal & Apples with Cinnamon	4.0
Beech Nut	Oatmeal & Apples	4.0

Above tables from: "Whoa Baby: Even Some Baby Food Is Acidic" by Dr. Jamie
(www.refluxcookbookblog.com)

pH of Baby Foods in Pouches and Jars
(Age 4–6 Months & Toddlers)

Brand	Description	pH
Earth's Best Jar	Summer Vegetable Dinner	5.7
Earth's Best	Squash Sweet Peas	5.3
Earth's Best Jar	Winter Squash	5.2
Earth's Best	Pumpkin & Spinach	5.0
Earth's Best	Sweet Potato & Beets	4.9
Earth's Best Jar	Sweet Potato & Chicken Dinner	4.9
Earth's Best	Butternut Squash	4.7
Happy Baby	Apricots, Sweet Potato	4.5
Happy Baby	Pears	4.5
Happy Tots	Blueberries, Yogurt, Oats, Chia	4.3
Happy Tots	Apples, Cinnamon, Yogurt & Oats, Chia	4.2
Happy Baby	Apples, Kale, Spinach	4.2
Earth's Best	Banana, Blueberry	4.2
Happy Baby	Pears, Peas and Broccoli	4.2
Happy Baby	Banana Beets & Blueberry	4.1
Earth's Best	Sweet Potato & Apple	4.1
Happy Tots	Sweet Potato, Carrots & Cinnamon	4.1
Happy Tots	Pears, Kiwi & Kale	3.9
Gerber Container	Pear, Pineapple	3.8
Happy Tots	Pears, Raspberries, Butternut Squash, Carrots	3.8
Happy Baby	Apples, Guavas, Beets	3.8
Earth's Best Jar	Apple, Apricots	3.7
Earth's Best Jar	Apples	3.6

Your Baby's Position

Other than dietary habits, there are some anatomical ways to aggravate or improve your baby's reflux. It's basic mechanics. Remember when your obstetrician suggested you begin sleeping on your left side or up on a bunch of pillows to alleviate your own regurgitation? This is because reflux can happen much more easily when a person is lying on his or her back. Because of the asymmetrical shape of the stomach, sleeping on one's left side helps the diaphragm pinch the LES closed. The American Academy of Pediatrics recommends that infants sleep on their backs (supine) to avoid sudden infant death syndrome (SIDS).[88] Consequently, positioning infants in any other way to alleviate reflux is not an option, with the exception of allowing them to sleep on their back but at an incline.

Babies who sleep on an incline with the head elevated may dramatically improve their reflux. There are many baby seats and similar products on the market to help keep the head/body elevated. Sometimes desperate parents may take their screaming child into the car for a calming drive. Parents have even been known to keep their baby in the car seat while in the house, rocking it as a last resort to keep the baby calm. Baby car seats, however, are not always effective for the purpose of relieving reflux because most position children with their legs higher than their chest, which increases pressure on the stomach, and can lead to more reflux.

New reflux-alleviating positioners come on the market frequently, so do your research and considering trying one of these products. However, you need to know that none of them is FDA approved, and the FDA actually warns against use of these products for infants due to possible Sudden Infant Death Syndrome (SIDS).[90] You can also check with your local children's hospital to see if it has any recommendations or concerns about specific products for this purpose. In any event, for babies suffering from reflux, sleeping at an incline may help.

Drinks

During the first year of life, the focus of infant feeding should be on breastfeeding or formula until about six months, at which point solid foods may be introduced in complement.

A 2017 study looked at trends of beverage consumption in infants and toddlers from the 0 to 24 month age group.[91] Researchers found that the average intake of all nutrients in the 0 to 6 months and 7 to 12 months age groups met dietary recommendations; however, in the older age group, 13 to 24 months of age, toddlers were consuming far too much cow's milk and fruit juice.[91,92]

National trends indicate that among toddlers one to two years old, the proportion drinking fruit juices was 51.8 percent in 2017.[91] Fruit juice (aside from being extremely acidic) leads to dental disease (cavities), obesity, and our nation's booming childhood type 2 diabetes epidemic.[91-94]

> ## No Juice for Babies: Too Much Sugar and Acid
> There is no reason a baby should be drinking juice, not even diluted.

When ready to drink from a cup, encourage your child to drink water in lieu of sugary drinks. By not exposing your child to sugar at such a young age, you can prevent them from developing a sugar addiction.

The American Academy of Pediatrics recommends a maximum of four ounces of juice, total, per day, for children between the ages of one and three years old.[93,94] The upper limit for children ages four to six is 4 to 6 ounces per day; the limit for children up to eighteen years of age is 8 ounces (1 cup) per day.[93,94] Our message: eat the fruit; don't drink fruit juices. This way, your child will incite a healthy metabolism by breaking down the nutrients and fiber in whole fruits instead of guzzling down excessive sugar and empty calories.

Feeding Too Late

The risk of acid reflux is increased depending on timing of eating and drinking relative to when we lie down. The digestive process, especially emptying of the stomach, takes four to six hours for adults and one and a half to two hours for infants. This means that after eating, it takes time until most of the food has been digested enough to leave the stomach and make it into the intestines, where the threat of reflux is low. We recommend that parents stop the bedtime bottle before their baby turns twelve months and begin developing a nighttime routine that involves finishing dinner, having a bath, reading a book, and going to bed.

Once babies turn twelve months old, the American Academy of Pediatrics recommends ending bottle feeding, because of the risk of tooth decay. Healthy babies usually do not need the extra calories before bedtime. When we suggest their child should stop having milk or any other snack at bedtime, most parents look at us with disbelief. Their first reaction is usually, "There is no way my kid will go to bed without milk!" But lying down with a full stomach will aggravate reflux. Remember, the distance from the stomach to the mouth in infants and toddlers is not very far, so any leftover stomach contents can easily come back up.

For years, we've asked every family what their child eats and drinks throughout the day, and specifically if they drink milk or eat a snack before going to bed. Almost always, parents report within days or a couple

> ### The Dairy Dilemma: Should Babies Drink Milk at All?
>
> Despite generations of advertising and the support of the USDA (U.S. Department of Agriculture), there is conflicting evidence that dairy products in general, and milk in particular, are healthy; indeed, there is some evidence that they are not.[13-18, 95-98] (Dr. Jamie personally does not eat any dairy products, and she and her family drink water.)

ot weeks of discontinuing bedtime snacks that chronic runny nose and congestion clear up.

What, How, and When to Feed

As your baby continues to grow, issues with spitting up and fussiness usually decrease, especially as baby cereal, mashed foods, and more solids are introduced. This begs the question: how early can a liquid diet be supplemented with solid food? What are safe foods to introduce into a baby's diet and in what order?

Reflux should get better as a baby grows and its digestive tract (esophagus, stomach, intestines) develops and matures. As a baby's diet gets more solid, the thicker and heavier food, weighed down by gravity, is more difficult to back up from the stomach into the esophagus and the throat.

The American Academy of Pediatrics recommends waiting until a baby is around six months of age to introduce solids (AAP.org). According to the AAP, "Introducing solids prior to four months of age is associated with increased weight gain and morbid obesity, both in infancy and early childhood." Later on, introducing your baby to a variety of textures and healthy foods is deemed as a good and healthy practice.

Vegetables and fruits are the most important solid foods to introduce. The earlier babies are exposed to healthy eating, the more likely they are to maintain a healthy diet later in life. Learning early on to identify high acid foods and snacks is beneficial to the whole family and will ensure reflux and its associated symptoms will not reappear during the school-age years and beyond.

Regarding snacks, the AAP recommends that after the nine-month mark, parents should offer two to three healthy snacks per day, preferably fruits and veggies. (From a reflux perspective, bananas, red apples, and melons are the least acidic fruits.) The AAP also recommends maintaining fruit and vegetable consumption after finger foods are introduced. Note: For many children, this is the age when there can be a decrease in fruit and veggie consumption and an increase in non-healthy and non-nutritious finger and snack foods, such as crackers, french fries, cereal, and cookies— this stage requires parental monitoring and intervention.

As discussed at the beginning of this book, processed foods are unhealthy. When parents grab puffed snacks, goldfish crackers, or other fun, crunchy packaged foods, their baby or toddler is digesting unnecessary acids, fats, and sugars—all culprits in loosening the LES in the esophagus—which can lead to or exacerbate reflux. Learning early that these foods should not be go-to snacks can help your child stay healthy today and later on in life.

Making Low-Acid Baby Food, Stage by Stage

We hope that the discussion and listing of the pH levels of processed baby foods whether in jars, cans, or pouches has given you pause, especially if your child suffers from reflux. What then, should you feed your child? Whole plant-based foods are the answer. When looking for what type of baby food to give your child, think about preparing the baby-mush at home, using whole, unprocessed foods.

Why buy jarred applesauce, when you can make your own? Want to experiment with sweet potatoes or graduate to giving your baby mashed bananas? These options are easy enough to make on your own, instead of buying packaged acidified (and expensive) versions. If you are able to make the time and devote the energy necessary to make your own baby food, the advantage will be full control over what your baby is eating.

Be sure that you are safely preparing the food and that its texture and consistency is appropriate for your baby. Consider how the brand baby foods often indicate a "stage" or eating level on the label, from smooth one-ingredient foods (like peas) to chunkier, mixed recipes (chicken noodle) for more advanced eaters. Be sure to discuss with your child's doctor how to safely prepare and store your homemade products.

If you do not have the time to prepare your own baby food, look for jarred food that is natural, sugar-free, BPA-free, and made with few preservatives. As a rule of thumb, you want the first ingredients listed on the label to be the whole foods you are looking for. Ingredients are listed in the order of the amount each jar contains. (Refer to our list of baby foods and their pH levels on pages 28–30.)

Stage 1: (6 to 8 months)

Stage 1 baby food is for children about six to eight months of age, or whenever they begin to lose the "tongue thrust" reflex, which is important for sucking the breast/bottle when they are young.

Stage 1 food is the first solid food a baby experiences. Therefore, it should be thinly pureed and not include a combination of food types, as you need to be sure that your baby is tolerating each food product with no allergic reaction. Included in this group are: carrots, green beans, peas, sweet potatoes, butternut squash, winter squash, avocado, red apples, bananas, pears, plums, peaches, prunes, and pumpkin. The AAP recommends starting with cereal and then moving on to vegetables and possibly meats (pureed) to encourage non-sweet appetites.

Note: Peas and beans are tough to puree and may be labor intensive because the skin needs to be peeled and the veggies prepped. You may consider holding off on peas and green beans until your baby is a bit older and can snack on them as finger foods.

Stage 2: (8 to 10 months)

Stage 2 baby food is given to babies who have mastered stage 1 and are ready for thicker food. This food group is still supposed to have a low allergy potential and should have a high protein content. Stage 2 foods include cereals, lentils, eggs, blueberries, small wheat-based pasta, yogurt, and melons (honeydew, cantaloupe, watermelon). Examples include mashed bananas and mashed avocado. Yogurt-based food that you can prepare at home can be yummy as well.

Stage 3: (9 to 10+ months)

This stage of food provides a chunkier consistency and is usually introduced around nine months of age after a child has mastered stage 2 food. Stage 3 foods include oatmeal, grains, baby pasta, and cut-up pancakes that you can prepare at home. Stage 3 can incorporate yogurt and various fruits. Puree fruit and blend it with plain almond milk.

Stage 4: (Graduate!)

When babies are able to sit in a high chair and hold their heads upright and have some teeth, they may be ready to eat more solid foods, as long as the foods are cut into very small pieces. Examples of stage 4 foods include pasta, cooked soft veggies, such as carrots, zucchini, peas, and tiny pieces of meat.

How to Make Your Own Baby Food

You will need a food processor, blender, or "bullet" of some kind. (Note that most of the time, you will have to boil, steam, or microwave the fruits and veggies to soften them before blending.) Combinations that babies love are cooked carrots with spinach, apples and/or beets, blueberries with banana, kale and/or avocado, zucchini with spinach, sweet potato and/or pear, banana with tofu, pumpkin, and dates. If you need a liquid to soften the consistency, we recommend using almond milk. Note: all of these recipes can be augmented with flavorful "seasonings" like ginger, cinnamon, thyme, basil, or even orange zest. In addition, you can mix or match any of the above items to find your own baby's favorite recipes. (If you can afford to do so, buy organic.)

When thinking about what to prepare for your young child, see the shopping lists in Chapter 6 and Appendix D to find low-acid fruits, veggies, and other products and experiment with various combinations.

Always consult with your pediatrician to see when your baby is ready to advance to the next stage and which food items to avoid or introduce. Remember that the following foods are choking hazards in young children and should be avoided: grapes, any type or shape of hot dogs, nuts, and hard candy. For more information, see "Foreign Bodies" in Appendix B: It May Not Be Reflux, pages 183–184.

We hope that this chapter has raised your antennae to the possibility that your baby might have reflux, and that reflux control can be achieved most of the time without medical intervention. Key measures to improve your baby's outlook include a low-acid diet, avoidance of other reflux-causing foods such as processed meats, cheese, and fast food, and no bottle or feeding in or before bed. Also, remember, we anticipate that you will consider adjusting the dietary habits of your whole family for the benefit of your child.

CHAPTER 4

Children Two to Twelve

I t's hard to imagine, but the next decade of your child's life is about to hit warp speed. Your toddler will go from potty training to Little League to fractions quicker than you can say "growth spurt." After infanthood, navigating your child's health and nutrition becomes interspersed with new complexities, such as school, peer pressure, scheduling, and many other outside influences and distractions that may make you nostalgic for the days of bottles and diapers.

From now on, your child will be out in the world, experiencing things beyond your control, like processed foods, other people's habits and routines, dietary options at daycare and school, as well as the biggie: exposure to more germs than ever! In fact, as ear, nose, and throat doctors (ENTs), we meet parents and families of children every day who are referred to us because their children seem like they are "sick all the time" with ear infections, runny or stuffy noses, recurrent strep, tonsillitis, chronic cough, or a cough and raspy voice that sound remarkably similar to that of a cigarette smoker!

Generally, it's obvious when your child is actually sick, such as when a fever accompanies a runny nose, cough, diarrhea, vomiting, decreased appetite, or disrupted sleep. If the symptoms persist, you may be told by a doctor that your child has a "sinus infection" and/or ear infection. In the two- to six-year-old age group, doctors will often prescribe allergy medications like nasal steroid sprays, or antihistamines, or asthma treatments. The key is to recognize that although your pediatrician may have prescribed nebulizers to treat "asthma" or other medications for presumed "allergies," the symptoms may not go away.

We have observed that for thousands of children, these symptoms occur not just when the child is suffering from a cold, but every day. Many parents may also describe a rattle in their child's chest, a sound that suggests phlegm (mucus) stuck in the back of the throat that can't be coughed out. In this situation, when the child has no fever, has a normal appetite, and is able to go to daycare or school and participate in normal daily activities—but always with a cough, runny nose, and nasal congestion—the real culprit may be respiratory reflux.

Reflux looks and feels very different in children than it does in adults and teens. Often children do not feel or report symptoms of heartburn as one might expect. Because they are not aware of these symptoms and may often not communicate that backwash is coming up into their throats, we characterize these children as suffers of "silent reflux." They can exhibit ear, nose, and throat complaints as well as breathing issues that are mistakenly diagnosed as "asthma" or "allergies," when in reality, most of these symptoms are triggered or made worse by respiratory reflux.

Some children have the ability to tell adults that their food or stomach content has come back up into their throat. A parent once reported that her child's Montessori school principal had called because her three-year-old complained that her lunch had come back up! Upon further questioning, the mother revealed she was packing what she considered a "balanced" lunch for her daughter, consisting of a fruit punch drink, a peanut butter and jelly sandwich, and Oreo cookies! A typical lunch like this is, in fact, loaded with things that cause acid reflux!

So, what are the differences between being sick all the time and reflux-related respiratory issues associated with a "bad reflux diet"? Discussed below are some symptoms caused by acid reflux that may mimic other illnesses.

Reflux Symptoms

Dry swallows. If you notice your child is swallowing when s/he is not actually eating or drinking, we refer to the behavior as "dry swallows." This may be a sign that stomach contents have traveled back up past the upper esophageal sphincter and that your child is swallowing down the backwash (yes, pretty gross, and probably not so tasty). Dry swallowing from acid reflux can also occur when a child is sleeping.

Decreased interest in eating solid food at meals. Many healthy children may start refusing to eat table foods that they previously liked or have eaten in the past and favor softer items like yogurt and pudding. Sometimes, they will continue to drink milk and other beverages, especially if these drinks are sugary. Acid reflux can cause discomfort or even pain when swallowing or cause a child to feel like there is something stuck in the back of their throat.

Bad breath that either smells like sour milk or vomit. This odor may be due to fermented milk or partially digested food refluxed into the swallowing tube (esophagus) or into the throat or mouth.

Frequent awakening during the night. Reflux can cause middle-of-the-night awakening. Often, parents remark that their child seems to be unusually congested during these episodes. Reflux of stomach contents can cause the body to dry swallow backwash, which may awaken a sleeping child. Coughing can also occur during sleep to protect and clear the airway of acid reflux. Nasal congestion related to reflux can make it harder to breathe through the nose and more difficult for a child to sleep peacefully through the night.

Frequent vomiting when there are no other symptoms that suggest acute illness, such as fever. If your child seems to throw up more often than normal, think reflux, and talk to your child's doctor to discuss whether referral to an ENT or GI specialist is necessary.

Complaints that food and liquids come back up into the throat. This can occur immediately or up to an hour after eating. The more sugar, fat, fried foods, and foods rich in cream and dairy that are consumed, the more likely stomach contents will be difficult to digest, which leads to increased reflux.

From the Case Files of Dr. Karen

A parent reported that her seven-year-old kept complaining of pain in her chest, which caused immediate concern regarding a possible heart condition. The child's doctor quickly ruled out that possibility with an ECG (electrocardiogram). Upon further questioning about any changes in dietary habits, the mother recalled that she recently bought several cartons of chocolate milk (since it was on sale) and that her daughter loved it. The chest pain turned out to be a symptom of acid reflux! The child was also found to be sensitive to lactose.

Shortness of breath, especially during sports activities. This can be a scary reflux symptom. If an otherwise healthy child gets easily winded and needs to sit out in the middle of a practice, routine, or game, and the "asthma" medication your doctor has already prescribed is not working, reflux may be the cause. Always ask yourself what your child ate or drank within an hour before practice (or during breaks) and if there are sweet snacks and juice, fast foods, or other items high in sugar and acid involved. There is a chance that acid reflux is causing your child's airway to constrict by triggering a tightening in the throat or lungs, mimicking the symptoms of "asthma."

Chronic cough, day or night, even when a child doesn't have a cold. This is a complicated issue and can be cough-variant asthma or chronic inflammation of the mucous membrane in a child's sinus cavities; however, more commonly, the cough is due to reflux.

Frequent stomach aches. While there are many causes of stomach upset or stomach pains, we have observed that in children who have chronic or frequent constipation in tandem with an unhealthy diet, acid reflux is the culprit. These children tend to complain of stomach issues and often get referred to a GI specialist for evaluation.

Take stock of your child's diet. We have observed that many toddlers drink very little water, instead favoring chocolate or strawberry milk, along with other sugary beverages like lemonade, fruit punch, pouched drinks, and sports drinks. In addition, preschool-aged children often love and consume too much dairy (with their parents' encouragement) in the form of sugary pudding and processed yogurt products. Today's children consume a diet high in sugar and dairy, comprised of mostly processed foods instead of fresh and natural produce high in fiber and healthy nutrients.

The Acid Reflux Aliases in Children

In the last chapter, focused on newborns to two-year-olds, we introduced the concept of acid aliases: symptoms that look like one thing, "allergies," "asthma," "croup," or congestion, but are really acid reflux in disguise. In our experiences, we have found five common acid aliases with which children are frequently misdiagnosed, and therefore, have not yet discovered the proper treatment for: asthma, noisy breathing, congestion, allergies, and chronic cough.

The Asthma Alias

Almost every child we have seen presenting a chronic cough has already been prescribed breathing treatments and inhalers for "asthma." Of course, there is a legitimate diagnosis called cough-variant asthma, in which a cough is the primary symptom instead of wheezing, but this is often a misdiagnosis. For most children between the ages of one and six, the cough first starts after a viral illness, like a cold, but while the runny nose eventually dries up and the fever subsides, the cough persists.

Asthma, as in many other medical diseases, may be explained as a condition with the underlying cause of inflammation. In this case, the smooth muscles that control the opening and narrowing of the airway in the lungs may be reactive to a trigger and constrict, making it harder for a patient to breathe.

The medical test most often used to diagnose asthma is to have patients undergo what's called a pulmonary function test. For this test, the patients are asked to blow as hard and as fast as they can into a machine. An inhaler is used to dilate (open up) their airways, and after a few minutes, the patients again blow into the machine. To detect if a patient has asthma, doctors compare test results before and after the administration of the inhaler. In order to be able to perform this test, however, generally a child needs to be about age six or older. It can be incredibly difficult to have a preschooler sit still and blow into a machine in order to diagnose asthma. Preschoolers are unable to do pulmonary function tests and cannot accurately be diagnosed until they are older.

Another method to diagnose asthma is, more simply, for doctors to use their stethoscopes and listen to the child's chest. Wheezing is the sound most descriptive of asthma. When the airways in the lungs are restricted by asthma, a patient will wheeze and/or cough on exhalation.

Sugar is a trigger for inflammation that restricts breathing. Children with a diet that is excessively high in sugar from processed foods and beverages are likely to experience high acidity in their stomachs, putting them at risk for respiratory reflux, which can trigger cough and asthma-like symptoms. Our patients who suffer from asthma severe enough that they require daily breathing treatments on a scheduled basis almost always have improved symptoms, with fewer attacks and episodes after switching to drinking mostly water, cutting out sugary drinks and processed snack foods, and eliminating bedtime snacks.

You may be asking at this point, "So how do I know if my child really has asthma?" Good question. We propose that you first focus on your child's diet and what he or she eats and drinks throughout the day (refer to the "Bad Reflux Diet" Quiz on page 13) paying a great deal of attention to the timing of the last meal of the day and the consumption of drinks other than water, especially in the evening. If you know that your child is not consuming excessive dairy or sugar and drinks mostly water, but still has problems like wheezing, you and your child's doctor can probably rule out reflux as a cause for these symptoms.

Asthma: In or Out?

When diagnosing asthma, the first question a physician (or a parent for that matter) should ask is whether the difficulty breathing occurs when breathing in or out or both. Generally, difficulty breathing in is due to reflux, and trouble breathing out is due to asthma. In our experience, more than half of children with "asthma" actually have respiratory reflux. True asthma is not just any kind of noisy breathing; it is trouble getting the air out of the lungs during expiration that produces a wheezing noise.

The Noisy Breathing Alias

There are a variety of noises children can make when they breathe. Take a nice slow deep breath through your nose. Notice that when we breathe in, everything opens up so that air can flow into our lungs without excessive work: the chest increases in size, our vocal cords relax, and the diaphragm moves downward. Noise that occurs when a child is breathing in (inspiration) generally means there is blockage in the airway somewhere up high, above the vocal cords.

Noises that occur when a child is breathing out (expiration) generally mean that the narrowing is likely below the vocal cords in windpipe (trachea), the lungs or in the lower chest, and are much more likely to represent asthma. As you sit now and breathe out slowly, feel the air being gently pushed out of your body. Your diaphragm and the smooth muscles that control your lungs are contracting to narrow the airway and push the air out of your body.

Try to whistle with your mouth wide open. You won't hear any sound until you narrow your lips so that airflow becomes turbulent and constricted; only then will you create the whistling sound. The same goes for a child with unusually loud breathing, whether awake or asleep. Something is causing the airway to narrow so that air has to rush out of a tighter space. This turbulent airflow creates a loud noise others nearby can hear. Some types of abnormal noises that children can make are as follows:

Stridor. Stridor refers to noisy breathing. Stridor on the inhalation is not rare in babies. The most common reasons for young babies to make this noise are reflux and laryngomalacia ("floppy" structures above the vocal cords leading to premature closure of the voice box upon inspiration). It is possible that stridor will still occur in toddlers, but generally, by preschool age, children have grown big enough for the sound to become rare. If you detect stridor in your child, talk to your doctor and discuss the option of a referral to a pediatric ENT doctor for further evaluation.

Biphasic (Both In and Out) Stridor

Biphasic stridor is characterized by very noisy breathing when a child is both inhaling and exhaling. This indicates to an ENT that something—either a foreign object or a viral illness causing swelling in the subglottis, the area below the vocal cords—is constricting the passage of air. Usually these children will have a bark-like cough or what is called croup, laryngotracheobronchitis. If observed, speak to a doctor immediately and/or go to an emergency room. Make sure that no one who cared for the child witnessed any choking episode in which your child may have put food or a foreign object in their mouth and inhaled or swallowed it. Foreign objects can be a cause for significant noisy breathing and respiratory distress and require immediate medical attention, preferably at a children's hospital emergency department. (See also "Foreign Body in the Airway," page 183.)

Stertor or "piggy noises" like the snorting of a pig. Stertor is the sound one makes when the nasal passages are obstructed by mucus. As a child tries to breathe through the nose, vibrations in the soft palate in the back of the throat create a fluttering, congested noise. When parents hear this, they often want the child to blow their nose or cough to clear away the phlegm, because it may sound like there is a lot of mucus in the head.

"Darth Vader" breathing. Like the famous villain, you can hear this child breathing from quite a long distance away! Such a child is not in any distress, meaning they are not struggling to breathe and are still active and happy. This sound is not the same as wheezing, but a sign that there is not enough space in the upper airway for air to pass through. Children who sound like Darth Vader and breathe with their mouths open usually have enlarged adenoids that limit space for air to flow. Acid reflux by itself can cause nasal congestion and, in turn, loud breathing, but more often, Darth Vader noises usually stem from enlarged tonsils and/or adenoid tissues.

Wheezing. Wheezing occurs when the small airways or bronchioles in the lungs are constricted. Most parents we see describe any noise they hear from the child's mouth as wheezing, which usually elicits a response of concern for true asthma. Asthma-related wheezing that is loud enough for someone to hear without putting a stethoscope to the chest of a child indicates a very severe asthma attack that requires immediate attention. Acid reflux can trigger constriction and tightening of the small airways that lead to wheezing or recurrent and chronic wheezing episodes, but the previously described breathing sounds should be considered as well. It is important to know that respiratory reflux is also a common trigger for true asthma.

The Congestion Alias

Thousands of children of various ages come to our clinics suffering from chronic congestion or stuffy noses. What's most concerning to us as ear, nose, and throat specialists is the tendency of doctors to blame a little nose that doesn't work on either "allergies" or a "sinus infection."

Let's talk about congestion and how the parts inside the nose cause the blockage of airflow that makes your child sound like s/he has a cold: There are there three paired structures (rarely four) inside the nose called turbinates. Imagine three shelves in each side of the nose, covered with the living tissue of the nose, which, itself, contains microscopic little hairs (cilia) that help the nose keep itself clean.

When we have a cold or allergies or when women are pregnant and under the influence of estrogen, the living tissue or mucosa in the nose can swell to take up space so that less air can flow through. When there is swelling of the mucous membrane, it may come with discharge of clear mucus and the wet congestion of a runny nose. Other factors that can cause wet congestion include rapid changes in temperature, such as, going into a cold, air-conditioned space after being outside on a sunny summer's day, or eating hot or spicy food, what we call vasomotor rhinitis.

Children are often congested without truly being sick. In fact, while most parents and even doctors may blame congestion and runny nose on "allergies" or germs at daycare, what is commonly the cause of a misbehaving nose is acid reflux and issues related to digestion and constipation.

Do you remember the most recent time you were sick and vomited or accidentally gagged yourself while brushing your teeth? As soon as our gag reflex is activated and any reflux or retching occurs, the eyes immediately start to tear up and the nose becomes congested with clear mucus.

Children often have reflux all night long if they go to bed with undigested foods. As the parasympathetic nervous system in the body is activated by reflux, nasal congestion occurs that can cause snoring and mouth breathing during sleep.

The Chronic Cough Alias

Chronic cough is likely the most frustrating symptom for most parents and doctors, including ENTs, because there is no medication or operation with which to cure it. Reflux is the most common cause of chronic cough in children (and in adults, too[3]).

Cough is an important reflex that the body has designed to protect our airways. Cough is not always a sign of asthma but is often assumed to be. Reflux will trigger the body to protect itself from the material entering the lungs. The body protects the airway the only way it knows how: by coughing repeatedly. When coughing, either as a reflex or on purpose, we force air to flow outwards at up to 100 miles an hour! As air rushes out of the lungs and through the windpipe the obstruction is projected away from our airway. A body that is frequently having this issue will react with chronic cough. In children, sugary beverages and food and dairy products can lead to reflux and daily cough.

The Croup Alias

Croup, also known as "laryngotracheobronchitis," is inflammation of the mucous membranes of the entire airway from the voice box, down the windpipe, all the way to the lungs. When the mucous membranes of the airways are inflamed and swollen, a child's breathing passages become constricted. As air is pushed forcefully out by the diaphragm against a semi-closed voice box, built-up pressure causes the voice box to suddenly open and air to come rushing out. As air rushes through this narrow area we hear it as a "barky" or "croupy" cough. This may also coincide with a raspy voice.

Most doctors are taught only one explanation for croup: that it is caused by a virus, and must be treated with steroids. We have, however, in practice, observed many children who suffer from recurrent "croup" without actually being sick! Usually there is sudden onset of barky cough in the middle of the night, no fever the day before, and no other signs of illness. In this case, acid reflux is causing the inflammation that results in "croup." These attacks can be very scary in young children, and it is extremely worrisome for parents to watch their child struggling to breathe. If your child has a barky cough in addition to trouble breathing or labored breathing, take your child to an emergency room without hesitation.

From the Case Files of Dr. Jamie: Recurrent Croup

A five-year-old obese girl presented with recurrent croup. She would awaken from sleep once or twice a month gasping for air with a croupy cough. Usually, these episodes would last less than a few minutes, but on occasion, they lasted for hours. For this reason, she was admitted to the emergency room for observation and treatment four times in one year. Additionally, the girl was on asthma medications including an inhaler; however, when an attack occurred, the inhaler didn't help. Dr. Jamie took a detailed history of the girl, including a dietary history. The girl's eating habits were unhealthy, dominated by sugary beverages, fast foods, cereals loaded with sugar, and excessive amounts of ice cream and cookies. Each night included a sugary bedtime snack. Dr. Jamie intervened by educating the parents on how to improve their child's diet, which included consuming more fruits and vegetables, and no bedtime snacks. Soon, the "croup" attacks ceased.

As a bonus, over time, the girl also lost a lot of weight.

The Allergy Alias

"Not all that runs is allergic!" There is not a single day in the clinic that we as ENTs don't meet at least half a dozen children of all ages with symptoms of nasal congestion and "allergies." Parents who believe that their children have allergies are baffled when allergy medications don't work. When we ask families how they know their child has allergies, we typically discover that they haven't been tested by an allergist, but simply put on allergy medications by their pediatricians.

While babies can be born allergic to foods or animals, rarely are they born already allergic to trees, grasses, pollen, dust mites, mold, and other allergens from the environment. Usually, environmental allergies occur after several years of repeated exposure. Having either or both parents with a positive allergy history can increase the risk of a child developing allergies later in life. For babies who have true allergies to cow milk protein (casein), signs may include bloody stool, bloating, and other gastrointestinal symptoms.

Many children, having suffered weeks and months of congestion and runny nose in the absence of fever or other signs of true illness, likely have reflux. After thousands of interviews over the course of our careers, we have observed that most often, what these children have in common is the habit of drinking milk and/or juice multiple times throughout the day and at bedtime. This is because our diet and the timing of what we eat and drink play a major role in how much acid enters our body and how those levels affect our bodily functions.

We Are What We Eat and When We Eat It

A twelve-year-old boy had complaints of chronic cough and shortness of breath despite treatment for "asthma." He was on the track-and-field team and hated always finishing last because of his labored breathing. After taking a detailed dietary history, it was obvious to us that he was drinking too many sugary soft drinks and was enjoying frequent bedtime snacks. After reducing excessive sugar in his diet and cutting out snacks within an hour and a half to two hours of bedtime, the boy began to feel much better and no longer experienced shortness of breath when running. Now, he often leads the pack during races and frequently places near the top.

Could it be as simple as that? Could what was thought to be asthma or reactive airway disease (RAD) really be due to what this boy ingested? The adage goes: "You are what you eat," and we couldn't agree more. In fact, we wish more medical doctors were well-versed in the importance of diet and nutrition, but the reality is that medical schools still dedicate little time to teaching nutrition in the curriculum of medical students. (See our Letter to Physicians on page xvi.) Reflux occurrence is determined by what we put into our bodies. Taking control of your child's health is all about understanding that what we eat, and when we eat it, determines how well our body performs.

Have you tried to talk while drinking something and either swallowed "wrong" or choked, and then coughed and coughed until you turned purple? Have you ever noticed that some beverages are more likely to trigger your cough than others? If so, we'd bet that those foods and drinks are meat, dairy, sugar, wheat, processed foods, and alcohol, because they are most prone to irritate the throat and airways. By design, our stomachs are filled with natural acids that are necessary for digestion, but when children eat or drink foods and beverages that are acidic, the additional acid causes a buildup, which has to go somewhere, and usually that somewhere is up into the airways!

Soft Drinks Are a Problem

Soft drinks are the poster child for the reflux epidemic. When children drink soda, they consume huge quantities of sugar, high-fructose corn syrup (HFCS), and acid. Moreover, the bubbles in carbonation expand in the stomach to make subsequent reflux all the more likely.[99]

No other single consumable item has had more influence on the decline of America's health than soda (although fast food is a close contender). Coca-Cola was invented in 1886, but it wasn't until World War II that Coke became "America's drink." In 1952, the first diet soda pop on the market was Kirsch No-Cal Ginger Ale; however, the largest increase in soda consumption in the United States started in 1965, when canned soda began to be distributed through vending machines.[1] In 1966, the National Soft Drink Association was formed (now the ABA, American Beverage Association) to lobby for the soft drink industry. The ABA has proven to be a well-funded and powerful adversary to healthy eating and drinking. While soft drinks remain a serious health risk, public advocacy has helped the consumption of soft drinks to decrease by about twenty percent in recent years.

In 1967, high-fructose corn syrup was introduced to the American marketplace. This form of sugar changed the glycemic index (sugar conversion), effectively increasing the sugar content of not only beverages but also many foods. A 20-ounce bottle of soda contains the equivalent of approximately 15 to 18 teaspoons of sugar (240 calories), and sugar-sweetened beverages are the single largest source of sugar in the American diet.[100-102] The average American drinks nearly 42 gallons of sweetened beverages a year, the equivalent of 39 pounds of extra sugar. Over the past thirty years, soda consumption has doubled and diabetes rates have tripled.[101]

Is diet soda any better? While it does not contain sugar, diet soda is still very unhealthy, because the sugar is being substituted by artificial sweeteners like aspartame (NutraSweet and Equal), sucralose (Splenda), and saccharin. Studies reveal that diet soda consumption is associated with weight gain, headaches, and depression.[10-11] The reason for the weight gain is unclear; however, like sugar, artificial sweeteners appear to trigger insulin release that drives fat storage. Ironically, when people drink diet soda, they may feel entitled to eat more food. Incidentally, aspartame is found in thousands of other products besides soft drinks.

The Glycemic Index

The glycemic index (sugar conversion) is a way to think about sugars in carbohydrate foods and how much and how quickly your body's sugar level increases based on what you eat. The higher the glycemic index of the item, the worse it is for your body. For example, a glycemic index of 55 or less is considered low (good). A number of 70 or higher is considered high (bad). Depending on what you eat and how you prepare your food, the glycemic index may change. The more natural the food and the less processed, the lower the glycemic index.

It's 6:00 p.m.—Do You Know Where Your Dinner Is?

The risk of acid reflux also increases depending on the timing of eating and drinking relative to when we lie down. Typically, the digestive process requires about four hours in teens and adults and an hour and a half to two hours for younger children. This means that after eating, it takes hours until most food has been digested enough to leave the stomach and travel into the intestines. (For a refresher on the science of reflux and digestion, see pages 8–9.)

On intake, we ask every family what their children eat and drink throughout the day, and, specifically, if they drink milk or eat a bedtime snack. Parents of children ages two to twelve report that within days or weeks of increasing the time between eating and sleep, their child's chronic runny nose, "allergies," breathing problems, and congestion subside. We'll talk much more about high-acid foods and poor eating schedules next, but in short, we suggest trying to eat dinner no later than 6:00 p.m.

Unfortunately, with our busy grown-up lives and similarly over-packed schedules for our children, sitting down together at mealtime might seem an afterthought or a luxury. Imagine talking, chewing slowly, and enjoying a family meal without the presence of electronic devices and distractions—a pipe dream, right? Believe us when we say it is possible.

In order for our children to follow our advice as role models, we must first demonstrate positive behaviors. The entire family—adults and children regardless of age—needs to practice healthy eating habits and patterns and learn together how to make smart dietary choices. Remember, while our book is focused on the undiagnosed epidemic of acid reflux in children, unhealthy eating results in many other serious medical consequences. For example, chemicals found in soda have been shown to lead to osteoporosis (decrease in density of bone), insulin resistance, and diabetes.[99-102] Moreover, years of acid reflux can lead to damage that can increase risk of esophageal cancer.

Perfection is not the goal, but progress is. It's never helpful to compare your family to another; all that matters is that you are doing the best you can to raise your awareness and implement incremental positive changes each and every day.

Social activities, school obligations, a harried work schedule, just to name a few challenges, are factors that affect our families' lifestyles and eating choices and keep us at risk for acid reflux. Humans are creatures of habit. Regardless of age, bad habits can be turned into good ones by first asking yourself what is important to you when it comes to mealtime and eating. Perhaps you were not raised with healthy eating habits, in which case, it's completely understandable that you may not have been provided with the information and tools to live a healthy life—until now, that is. If it's important to you that everyone eats breakfast and/or dinner together as many days and nights as possible, what will it take to make that happen? Here are some additional questions to consider as you head down the path toward positive change:

- Does your family currently have healthy eating habits? Is there room for improvement?

- Do you think that there may be too much sugar and processed foods/unhealthy foods in your current routine?

- Do you eat out more often than you would like, and, if so, is this working for you and your family?

- When your family eats out, do you tend to drink sodas, juices, lemonade, and splurge on foods high in calories, sugar, and fats and order more than what's really necessary or healthy?

- What messages have you been sending your children about food and eating habits? Are you setting good examples? Do you talk with your children about why it's important to make good, healthy choices?

- Who is doing the shopping, and what is going into the shopping cart?

- What factors are being considered when the shopper is deciding what goes into the cart?

- Are the items being bought simply restocking what is being consumed, and would you like to consider trying new foods and recipes?

- Who will be cooking? Will you alternate? Who does what each night of the week?

- What can be made on days off, so that during the week, dinners can come together quickly with reheating?

- What is the plan for tonight and tomorrow? What is the backup plan?

- What time is your family's last meal of the day?

- What items are needed in order to make healthier lunches for yourself and your children?

If we don't talk about it, we send a message to our children that it must not be important, and they will not learn to avoid the many foods and drinks that can make them sick.

The good news about bad habits is that they don't have to last a lifetime. All of the nutrition and lifestyle choices we urge you to make will result in a healthier and happier child. A child without acid reflux is a well-rested, energetic, and nutritionally educated child, poised to win the battle against bad health as s/he grows into teen years.

CHAPTER 5

Teens

I f you find yourself reading this section, it's possible that your teen has been complaining of discomfort or has been seeing a doctor for conditions such as asthma or allergies with little or no results. Likely, your child is suffering from symptoms of acid reflux, symptoms that can be resolved without medication with simple dietary adjustments. Undoubtedly, teenagers who grow up learning about healthy nutrition and lifestyle will be less likely to suffer from a multitude of health problems, reflux included.

Reflux and its risk factors in teens are similar to adults and quite different from those present in younger children. It's in the nature of teenagers to assert their independence and explore the world outside of their home (i.e., they know everything). This newfound freedom can be a problem for a refluxing teenager.

A key motivational component may be how often your teen feels sick and miserable because of their reflux. As with adults, teenagers with disturbed sleep, sinus disease, asthma, chronic cough, difficulty swallowing, heartburn, indigestion, and/or lung disease, are more likely to be inspired to change, that is, to fix their diets and beat their reflux.

As opposed to children, whom we call silent refluxers, because they can't communicate their symptoms, teens have the ability to articulate exactly how they are feeling and are able to be assessed more fully and accurately through the use of a reflux symptom index (RSI).[48] You can take it too and compare your scores.

THE REFLUX SYMPTOM INDEX© (RSI)
How do the following affect you? 0 = No Problem   5 = Severe Problem

Hoarseness or a problem with your voice	0	1	2	3	4	5
Clearing your throat	0	1	2	3	4	5
Excess throat mucous or postnasal drip	0	1	2	3	4	5
Difficulty swallowing food, liquids, pills	0	1	2	3	4	5
Coughing after eating or lying down	0	1	2	3	4	5
Breathing difficulty or choking episodes	0	1	2	3	4	5
Troublesome or annoying cough	0	1	2	3	4	5
Sensations of a lump in your throat	0	1	2	3	4	5
Heartburn, chest pain, or indigestion	0	1	2	3	4	5
						RSI

No single number definitively proves reflux. A person can have reflux even if the score is quite low, but a score of 15 or higher indicates a 90 percent chance.[1,4,48]

In teenagers and adults, the symptoms listed in the RSI are the most common indicators of reflux; however, as a result of reflux, teenagers and adults can also experience ear symptoms, nasal congestion, sinus problems, and lung diseases.

Teens are just as likely to be misdiagnosed with allergy, sinusitis, and asthma as younger children; however, they are more likely to be placed on adult medications with side effects and undergo unnecessary and painful surgeries than their younger counterparts.

From the Case Files of Dr. Jamie:
An Odyssey of Misdiagnoses

A seventeen-year-old high school student whose diet was dominated by fast food and weekend alcohol binge-fests began to experience heartburn, hoarseness, cough, post-nasal drip, nasal congestion, and sinus headaches. After two months of feeling lousy he saw his family doctor who diagnosed reflux and put him on 40 mg of Prilosec per day. A month later, the teen's symptoms were unimproved and he was referred to a gastroenterologist (GI). The GI performed an endoscopy that showed mild inflammation of the esophagus, so the doctor increased the boy's Prilosec dosage to twice a day.

Over time, the boy's symptoms, particularly his sinus symptoms, worsened, and the family doctor referred him to an ENT surgeon. The ENT diagnosed nasal septal deviation, nasal congestion, and sinusitis. A sinus CT scan on the boy's sinuses showed mucoperiosteal thickening and fluid in the left maxillary sinus (but no evidence of chronic sinus disease). The surgeon performed a nasal septoplasty, bilateral turbinate reductions, and a balloon sinuplasty.

After surgery, the boy's symptoms improved, but by the end of his second week post-op, he was back to where he had started. The ENT sent the boy to an allergist who did skin testing and informed the patient that he had allergies to dust mites, grass, and some tree pollens. The teen was then started on monthly allergy shots (with no benefit). Soon a new symptom appeared—sharp abdominal pain. Two weeks after the belly pain began, the boy was admitted to a hospital for evaluation. He underwent a second endoscopy and a CT scan of his abdomen. Both test results were normal. He then came to see Dr. Jamie.

Dr. Jamie diagnosed persistent severe reflux as the cause of all the symptoms except for the abdominal pain, which was a side effect of the Prilosec. Dr. Jamie put him on a "reflux detox" program—early supper, no alcohol, a healthy low-fat, low-acid diet, plus Zantac (ranitidine) before each meal and before bed. With this program, he rapidly improved, and over several months, Dr. Jamie was able to educate the teen about healthy living. Subsequently, the young man was able to beat his reflux and his "sinus" symptoms without any medication.

As the case above demonstrates, teens suffering from reflux face a diagnostic minefield on the path to proper treatment. GIs do not know how to diagnose and treat respiratory reflux; by design, they are simply far too laser-focused on the esophagus and stomach. The diagnosis of respiratory reflux requires an ENT doctor who is experienced in this area. Secondly, proton pump inhibitors (medications such as Nexium and Prilosec) hardly ever control respiratory reflux in and of themselves. Their most common side effects are abdominal pain and diarrhea. Anti-reflux surgery will often do little to make any difference in improving a patient's situation without the necessary dietary and lifestyle changes. Post-nasal drip, nasal congestion, and sinus-like symptoms are among the most common symptoms of respiratory reflux.

There are many reasons why teens are prone to develop reflux. Previously healthy teens are at risk to develop reflux because of peer pressure to eat in unhealthy ways, including opting for fast food, consuming alcohol, and eating late at night. The risk of reflux for teens may worsen as they grow older, stay up later, and spend more time away from home.

TOP 10 DIETARY AND LIFESTYLE RISK FACTORS FOR REFLUX IN TEENS

1. Late-night eating

2. Lying down after eating

3. Skipping meals

4. Overeating

5. Being overweight or obese

6. Alcohol consumption (Yes, you should ask about it anyway!)

7. Eating high-fat/deep-fried foods

8. Drinking too much coffee (caffeine)

9. Consuming canned or bottled beverages

10. Eating too much high-acid (citrus) fruit

Over the past few decades, most Americans have been eating their evening meals later than in the past. In general, people are keeping later hours. After school or work, they may be involved in exercising, shopping, cooking, playing sports, or engaging in social activities. Most people who eat late also tend to overeat, typically because the evening meal is their biggest meal of the day.

Eating Too Late is the #1 Risk Factor for Acid Reflux in Teens

In younger people, the stomach normally takes a few hours to empty after a moderately sized meal. In older adults or for those who have severe reflux, stomach emptying is often delayed by four to six hours. Bedtime snacks? Always avoid them as they dramatically increase the likelihood of nighttime reflux.

Skipping breakfast and/or lunch is also a big mistake, and one that occurs a lot in teenagers. Being famished after a long day leads to overeating at night. In addition to three square meals, we also recommend healthy snacks interspersed throughout the day. This approach provides the body and brain an even distribution of fuel all day long and decreases the need to binge in the evening.

Alcohol is a common risk factor for refluxers. Most refluxers can tolerate a moderate amount of alcohol (at a relatively early hour), but if a person goes to sleep drunk or with a buzz, they can be expected to reflux all night. For most people, alcohol, particularly late into the evening, is a huge risk factor for reflux. Alcohol actually makes the stomach valve (the lower esophageal sphincter) relax, leading to acid more easily escaping the stomach as reflux. If your teen drinks alcohol with friends and then stops late at night for a fast-food meal, reflux is almost guaranteed. Underage drinking is a serious problem with regard to driving and overall safety, but it is also a serious risk for causing reflux. By the way, the same is true for adults. A "nightcap" is about the worst thing you can do for your reflux.

Alcohol is not the only problem beverage. Almost everything in a bottle or can (except for still water) is acidified, so if your teen drinks soft drinks, soda, juice, seltzer, or energy drinks, this may exacerbate reflux and cause other health problems as well.[1-4,99-102] In 2010, the American Beverage Association reported that the 12-to-29-year-old group consumed almost a half a gallon of soft drinks a day![4] Teach your children and your whole family to drink water, and get soda and juice out of the house.

High-fat foods including fatty meats, dairy products, and all deep-fried foods facilitate reflux by causing the LES valve to relax. Stopping on his way home late at night for a cheeseburger, fries, and a Coke is, perhaps, the worst thing a refluxer can do. In any case, fast food is generally unhealthy, especially late at night. Our recipes (page 87–169) contain predominantly low-fat ingredients.

For teenagers, coffee is more in vogue than ever! Whether they sport a cup of Joe as a fashion statement, meet up with friends in a cafe, or drink cups and cups of caffeine to pull an all-nighter before the SATs, teens are drinking more coffee every year and are starting at a younger age. Too much coffee causes reflux. According to the American Dietetic Association, the number of teenagers drinking caffeinated beverages has tripled since the 1970s.[103]

Like fat, excessive caffeine causes the LES valve to relax. For this reason, we recommend one or two cups of coffee a day, with a maximum of three. Coffee, regardless of amount, is a reflux trigger food for about 25 percent of people. For those affected, even decaffeinated coffee will cause reflux. A healthy alternative for people who can't drink coffee but who want some caffeine in the morning is a cup or two of tea.

More Coffee for Your Teen?

A high school in Texas was the subject of an article for the food service director, which reported that the school had run a successful coffee shop within the school campus for three years and counting. Not surprisingly, the most popular beverages were the ones including frothy milk toppings and sweet and savory flavorings. At three-to-five bucks a pop, what school wouldn't want to capitalize on the teen coffee trend? And many schools are. Ask your child whether s/he has coffee at school and how much s/he is drinking per day.[103]

What, then, can people with reflux safely drink? The answer, as always, is water. Get into the habit. For children thirteen and older, eight to ten glasses of water per day (about two liters) should do the trick—more if the child is athletic or actively competing.

Highly acidic fruit, namely citrus, may also present a problem. Lemons, limes, oranges, and grapefruits should be consumed in moderation—a few times a week or less—as their acidity is too high for most people with reflux. The same goes for (acidified) fruit juices.

Being Overweight

Overeating is a rather obvious reflux cause: If the stomach is over-filled, it is more likely to spill over into other parts of the body. We recommend small meals and snacks and a concerted effort to try to consume three-quarters of your daily caloric intake before 6:00 p.m. This takes some real discipline and planning. (See Chapter 6: "Healthy Living," pages 59–83.)

Being overweight is particularly problematic if the belly (abdomen) is enlarged. When an overweight person lies down, the extra poundage resting on the abdominal wall actually pushes on the stomach. Overweight teens and adults with reflux need to sleep on an incline—the closer to forty-five degrees upright, the better. Our "lean, clean, green, and alkaline" diet will result in weight loss over time the natural way. More about that later.

Whole Foods for the Whole Family

This is your wake-up call. In order to combat reflux, we recommend that you and your whole family make the changes and sacrifices necessary to revolutionize how and when you eat. Healthy and unhealthy eaters in the same household don't mix well.

Even though your teen may seem MIA or busier than ever, your family is still a unit. Healthy eating should be a family decision and a family activity. But make no mistake about it, your family, especially your teen, is going to have to make some sacrifices, especially in the beginning. Schedules will need to be restructured, and grocery shopping will feel more a team effort. You'll find some great advice on smart shopping in Chapter 6: Healthy Living. You can't have a nutritionally educated teen if the rest of the family has terrible eating habits. Here are some overarching tips for building a healthy family:

- Try to have your evening meals at home and as close to the same time as possible every night. We recommend 6:00 p.m. or as early as possible after 6:00 pm.

- Teens should learn how to cook. This will keep them less dependent on fast food.

- Help your teen resist social pressure to eat too late, or at the very least, minimize how many times a week or month s/he does. Going out to a fast food restaurant after a late soccer practice is always a bad idea.

- It may seem obvious at this point, but don't keep junk food (including chips, cookies, ice cream, processed meats, and cheese) in the house. Plan meals and snacks in advance before heading to the grocery store.

The following chapter expands on these topics as we continue to create your family's anti-reflux diet.

CHAPTER 6

Healthy Living

Few have the time, luxury, or inclination to be a master chef at home; however, everyone, especially parents and caretakers, can make a conscious decision and commitment to develop new habits for healthy living and eating. Whatever your reality or the challenges you face, we believe there are solutions for you and your family.

Healthy Solutions

Healthy Solution #1. Make it a policy to try new fresh whole foods and recipes. Mix up your food patterns once in a while to keep eating healthily interesting. Kids are drawn to primary colors, which makes the freshest foods your friends. You can turn your child's plate into a rainbow of anti-reflux food that is not only delicious and satiating, but also beautiful to look at. Even if your child accepts only one, two, or three bites of a new food, exposure to new tastes and textures will help them to expand their palate. Quick tip: Bribery can work wonders!

Health Solution #2. Talk about why it's important to eat healthy foods and drink plenty of water. Children learn better when they are taught the meaning behind an action. Simply telling a child what to put in their mouth doesn't show the method behind the madness. Don't underestimate your child's ability to understand why they need to make good food and beverage choices. Believe it or not, when faced with sound logic and reasoning, your child will likely opt in.

Healthy Solution #3. Teach children the importance of eating meals at scheduled times, three times a day, with at least one or two meals with the whole family. If scheduled eating is not emphasized, children may develop the habit of grazing. As parents and adults, we may be enabling unhealthy eating behavior and habits for the sake of ease, including allowing children to eat whenever they want without paying proper attention to the value of enjoying meals as a family.

Healthy Solution #4. Don't believe that some calories are better than none. Parents, especially mothers, often justify offering treats and snacks high in dairy and/or sugar because their child is a "terrible" or "poor" eater. Unfortunately, pediatricians often reinforce the idea that thin or "picky" eaters should get any calories possible, whether they are good calories or not! We completely disagree with these recommendations. If there are truly medical problems concerning poor weight gain, a child should see specialists like gastrointestinal (GI) or endocrinology doctors to be tested, in order to rule out issues like malabsorption or endocrine (hormonal) problems that can result in poor growth. When children eat and drink whatever they want, whenever they want, their stomach doesn't have a chance to empty and can get quite bloated. The result is a child who isn't usually hungry at mealtime.

Healthy Solution #5. Eat sweets earlier. It's just not realistic to tell a family not to allow their child any sugary treats. Dessert has long been a parent's ace-in-the-hole in the battle over dinner. A favorite treat might even convince a wary child to try Brussels sprouts! We recommend that if a family wants their child to have a dessert or treat, to enjoy it together while at the table, right after dinner or offer it after school, well before dinner time. Whatever you do, don't have sweets before bedtime! (More on this topic at the end of this chapter.)

Healthy Solution #6. Take your child to the grocery store. We love seeing parents shopping with their school-age children, teaching them to pick out fresh fruit and produce. This is a great way to expose children in a fun way to new varieties of foods. As more and more of the typical diet contains pre-packaged processed items full of unnatural additives and preservatives, an entire generation of children and young adults will lack the nutritional literacy necessary to know how to select fresh fruits and vegetables!

While shopping with your child, engage and empower them by reading ingredient lists and food labels together. This is very useful when deciding what is healthy to buy, while reinforcing the "why" of eating well. A simple rule to go by is that if the majority of ingredients can't be pronounced, it's probably too processed to eat.

Healthy Solution #7. Let kids assist in the kitchen, and let them get messy. Young children love to help, whether it's cracking open an egg or mixing anything in a bowl. Take advantage of your younger children's love of water by asking them to wash fruits; have older ones help hull strawberries or cut and prep. Yes, prepping, cooking, and cleaning up will likely take longer with kids in the kitchen, but without giving children of all ages an opportunity to be involved, they will lose out on learning to put thought, enjoyment, and effort into healthy eating routines. Remember, not knowing how to prepare and enjoy home-cooked meals may lead to unhealthy eating habits and negative consequences later on in their lifetimes.

Healthy Solution #8. Healthy prep work is worth the effort. You don't have to go out hunting for your meat or grow your own vegetables to make a healthy dinner! Meal preparation and healthy cooking do not mean that everything has to be prepared from raw produce or be made from scratch. While, in a perfect world, that would be ideal, most of us do not live in that world.

In preparation for busy weeknights, we often carve out time on weekends to tenderize, marinade and grill skinless chicken breasts. Later on, we can reheat the chicken and, with the addition of romaine lettuce, croutons, and Caesar dressing, toss a simple and easy salad for our weeknight dinner. For an easy and delicious reflux-friendly marinade, see page 141.

Fresh mozzarella and tomatoes (add fresh basil) can transform quickly into insalata caprese anytime. Boil-to-eat pasta, found in the refrigerated section of the grocery store, with store-prepared or homemade pesto sauce can get dinner on the table in about fifteen minutes! When looking for canned or jarred red sauce, choose items that do not list tomato puree and sugar as the first two ingredients. Ingredients that boast whole tomatoes and no added sugar (or acid) are best.

When cooking at home, try to think about balance by making sure to include protein (which can be plant-based), cooked and/or fresh vegetables, fresh fruits, and some carbohydrates. Think ahead about what would be reasonable for your schedule. Perhaps, use a crock-pot or pressure cooker to help save time.

Be sure that your children are eating at an appropriate time and not waiting for the adults to get home for a late dinner. If there is not enough time between eating and bedtime, risk for acid reflux increases.

It's helpful to think about what foods or drinks have given you heartburn or reflux in the past and to ask your children how they feel after eating or drinking certain items. If you and your family can become more aware and identify how you feel based on what you eat, you can prep your home-cooked meals to include foods that make everyone feel better.

A Twelve-Point Program for Healthier Eating and Living

This plan is flexible. Feel free to choose which step to tackle first (all are recommended).

1. Clean out your refrigerator and cupboard, removing soft drinks and high-fat and high-sugar items.

2. Drink water in lieu of soft drinks or fruit juices. Always keep a pitcher of ice water on the table to serve with home-cooked meals.

3. Eliminate fast food as a family meal option.

4. If fast food is a must, pick healthier choices on restaurant menus, such as salads, grilled meats, and plain baked potatoes.

5. Stop bedtime snacks.

6. Limit or eliminate processed meats, including bacon, sandwich meats, hotdogs, hamburgers, sausage, etc.

7. Cook at home as frequently as possible (see our recipes, pages 87–169).

8. Serve healthy snacks, especially fresh fruits like red apples (green apples are more acidic), bananas, peaches, dates, figs, and pears. Crackers with plain hummus, nuts, crudités, etc., can help keep snacks interesting.

9. Avoid or limit sugary desserts or snack foods (processed pudding cups, apple sauce, donuts, Pop-tarts, highly processed sugary snacks, and so on).

10. Read nutrition food labels (see Appendix C, page 196) during grocery shopping, remaining aware of excessive fat, sugar, and chemicals in the items you choose.

11. Try to eat as many plant-based and natural foods as possible.

12. Plan ahead by writing out grocery lists and packing your own snacks and foods to take to events and when traveling.

How to Turn a Juice Junky into a Water Worshiper

Water is boring, clear, and has virtually no taste, and that's exactly why we need to drink it. The human body is made up of almost 97 percent water and has the incredible ability to self-regulate electrolytes for maximal function. By ingesting acidic, sugary substitutes and denying ourselves and our children good old H_2O, we are preventing our amazing bodies from functioning the way they are designed to function.

The kidneys are an incredible filtration system—they remove excessive sugar and caffeine as well as "flush" various toxins out of our bodies. Water is critical for kidneys to excrete toxins and byproducts in the form of urine. Thirst is our body's way of signaling us to take in more water, so that it can continue to function. Only water can truly quench thirst

It is not uncommon while taking patients' histories for us to ask how much water a child drinks throughout the day. The answers we receive are often astonishing but admittedly, at this point, predictable. Most children drink predominately juice and milk (mostly chocolate or strawberry flavored). Parents of two- and three-year-olds have admitted to allowing their children up to three to four cups (6 to 8 ounces per cup) of juice per day! All day long, preschool-age kids are given a variety of sugar-loaded "fruit juices." It's amazing how easily people are led to assume that the word "fruit" on the front of a box means healthy. From decades of combined professional experience, we can estimate with confidence that the number one juice consumed by American preschoolers is apple juice. Other favorites include white grape juice, followed by imitation fruit juices, a variety of pouched drinks, fruit punch, orange-flavored sodas, and sports drinks.

The sports drinks are particularly frustrating. A child would need to endure two-to-three hours of intense physical exertion to warrant electrolyte replenishment. Children do not need Gatorade, Powerade, or any other boost or energy drink. The chemical dyes and sugar content alone are reason enough to stay away. Older children who participate in intense, sweaty sports practices may benefit from a drink containing electrolytes but in moderation.

When we first share with families that their child's symptoms are from acid reflux triggered by sugary drinks like juice, the question often follows, "Then what will she drink?" Usually there is a brief, awkward pause, after which we simply state, "Water." The fact that it never entered their minds indicates that these parents had long given up on water as an alternative. It's not easy having these conversations. Nutrition and dietary habit counseling typically take up much more time than the fifteen minutes allotted for a scheduled appointment, but as doctors we must make time for what's truly important. If we don't have these conversations now, we fail to empower our children with the tools needed for a healthy future.

Our goal is to help parents become aware that their children may not be drinking enough water and inform them how to successfully make water their child's primary beverage of choice. If you have a child who drinks mostly juice and other sugary beverages, here are our recommendations to help her or him transition to drinking mostly water:

How Much Water Should Children Drink?

The amount of water kids need is variable depending on many factors, including age, weight, gender, activity level, and ambient temperature. Thirst is a natural instinct that helps us prevent dehydration, but we should not wait until we are thirsty to drink water. Your children may not be drinking enough water. The body is self-regulating, so the focus is not on how many ounces or glasses of water your child should drink but that water, plain water, is the main liquid they consume every day.[104]

---

1. Dilute each cup of juice with water. Start by diluting your regular pour by half, a third, or even just a tenth. Each time you pour juice into a cup, add a little more water to the juice until, eventually, your child is just drinking water. (Yes, your child will taste the difference! S/he will likely complain, because s/he will taste less sugar. Don't give in! It may take some time. Be patient.)

2. Cut back on the frequency of all non-water beverages. If your child is drinking juice four times a day, cut the frequency down to three, then two, then one. The American Academy of Pediatrics recommends no fruit juice for infants up to twelve months and no more than four ounces per day for children between the ages of one and six.[8]

3. Give water in any form—plain water, ice water (many children prefer ice), or water with an added slice of fruit. Water infused with any cut up fresh fruit can make drinking more fun and "pretty." Offer it to your children repeatedly, even if they won't take it at first.

4. Encourage children to play by adding cut up fresh fruit to ice water, creating their own unique concoctions. Let them stir the water and fruit around with a straw, and have everyone drink the same beverage at mealtime.

5. Serve water with a BPA-free plastic fun cup and straw.

6. Blending up fresh fruit is also a great alternative to sugary processed

drinks and can be fun for young budding chefs and teens who are looking for something sweet and filling. Children and teens love "smoothies," so try blending various fresh fruit together with almond milk, ice, and even some vegetables for a refreshing and naturally sweet treat.

7. Don't give up if you have a bad day. It's not about perfection; it's about fighting for your child's health one drop at a time.

We've had parents send us videos of their two-year-olds having temper tantrums when transitioning to water. An all-time favorite video is of a toddler kicking and screaming on the kitchen floor, throwing a sippy cup filled with water across the room in dramatic protest to an unexpected change from the sweet drink he was used to. Expect your child to protest. Remember why you will not give in. Hopefully soon your child will be drinking water without a fuss. Likely, s/he will never remember these brief unhappy moments—only you will!

Sugar Addiction

Did you know that obesity and diabetes were uncommon, especially in children, until fast food and processed sugary beverages became mainstays in the American diet? Currently in the US, children as young as age ten are being diagnosed with diabetes. No longer just a disease of adulthood, obesity continues to affect very young children.

Another risk to American health is the new manufacturing practices of commercial corn, meat, and breads. In fact, there is processed sugar in some form in almost everything your family eats. Sugar is added to breakfast cereals, soups, condiments, snack foods, breads, and on and on and on.[4]

In 2016–17, the US produced 385,778,000 metric tons of corn[105]— almost as much as the rest of the world combined. Corn is converted into all kinds of processed sugars and other products. Corn is also the major feed source for cows and other farm animals, so even your beef and poultry are sweetened up. High-fructose corn syrup (HFCS), or its derivatives, is in thousands of products and has made millions of Americans, young and old, addicted to sugar.[1,4,7,8,10-12]

Infants, toddlers, children, and adults become addicted to sugar in the same way. Sugar addiction is similar to addictions to nicotine, alcohol, and narcotics. While we all know that addictions to drugs are absolutely not acceptable for our children, most of us do not have the same level of alarm when it comes to sugar. But as we saw with the toddler who threw a sippy cup of water in protest, sugar withdrawal can be as dramatic as any other serious chemical dependency.

Research has shown that sugar exposure changes the chemistry of the brain, so much so that when a laboratory rat is exposed to sugar, the rat no longer wants cocaine![106] If you make sure your infants and toddlers are not exposed to juice in the first place, and instead, foster their palates with an appropriate amount of milk or water, they will most likely grow up with a healthy aversion to non-water drinks loaded with sugar, caffeine, and dyes.

Breaking your family's sugar addiction may be difficult, but the program that we recommend below is a step-wise approach. Start by eliminating the low-hanging fruit by giving up soda, juices, and other sugary beverages. Limiting sugary treats in the house and highly refined processed breads and baked goods is another great way to start. We highly recommend reading nutrition food labels to avoid buying anything that contains high-fructose corn syrup. All sugars and carbohydrates are not created equal. Focus on consuming natural sugars from natural foods as these carbohydrates are quite different from the ones found in a bag of pretzels.

Your children, and, perhaps, your whole family, probably have a sugar addiction. These sugars can come in the form of cane sugar, molasses, honey, brown sugar, sucrose, lactose, glucose, malt syrup, and high-fructose corn syrup. If you go into the cereal aisle at your local grocery store, you will find that nearly every breakfast cereal has sugar added, and if you look at the ingredients, some are made up of as much as 50 percent sugar/sweetener. The label may not say "cane sugar," but look for the other sugar substitutes mentioned above, including corn syrup, lactose, and molasses. (See also Appendix C: How to Read a Nutrition Fact Label, page 196.)

Another major source of dietary sugar is bread, a staple in the American diet. Bread or bread-like products, often consumed with each and every meal and in the form of snacks, are made mostly of sugar. The label, however, doesn't read "sugar." While bread today is not officially genetically modified, it is a product of hybridization, in which new wheat strains were selectively bred for commercial gain.[8] In 1970, Norman Borlaug won the Nobel Peace Prize for inventing a new kind of wheat that people thought would end world hunger. Borlaug's wheat, known as dwarf wheat (Triticum), is disease- and drought-resistant and increases yields ten-fold per acre.[4,8]

This is not the wheat (Einkorn) that our parents grew up eating. One big difference is the sugar content. The glycemic (sugar conversion) index of cane sugar, the stuff in your sugar bowl, is 59. The glycemic index of bread made with dwarf wheat is 72![8]

Today, bread products made with dwarf wheat are about all you can get in the supermarkets. In order to fully understand the magnitude of our sugar intake, consider that the sugar in the bread that we eat with breakfast, lunch, dinner, and in snacks is added to the sugar that is consumed when we drink juice, soft drinks, and other processed food products. This amounts to a great deal of sugar and can lead to sugar addiction—and needless to say, acid reflux![4]

IOur stomachs and intestines are naturally filled with millions of good bacteria, called normal flora, which we need in order to regulate not only our digestive systems but also our immune systems. When their digestive tracks are bombarded with too much sugar and acid, it's likely that the natural community of bacteria existing within the gut will undergo negative change. Reflux also alters the body's normal flora for the worse.

Seven Steps to Quit (or Reduce) Sugar Addiction

1. Get high-fructose corn syrup (HFCS) out of your children's diet. Reduce your child's intake of pasta, cookies, cakes, energy bars, doughnuts, and everything else that contains added sugar, especially HFCS.

2. When your children crave sugar, turn to healthy carbohydrates like fruit. During the first few weeks, their sugar craving might seem intolerable, but it can be satisfied by fruits such as figs, dates, bananas, and red apples. If your child must have a dessert after a meal, consider options that include fresh fruit in some form.

3. Instead of sugary breakfast cereals as part of your child's morning routine, consider "hot" foods like oatmeal, and add fresh fruit like bananas and dried fruit such as raisins. Savory foods like grits and muesli may also be options. Eggs, hash browns, and hot rice can also fit the bill. The three-egg omelet with lox (smoked salmon) seen on page 96 is an example of an excellent alternative breakfast that you can make at home or order in a restaurant.

4. Understand why soda is so bad for your child's health. Do not buy soda in any quantity (diet soda included). You can even "digest" a cut of raw meat by pouring soda on it! Imagine how badly this acidity can hurt us once it's inside our bodies!

5. You can satisfy your child's craving for carbohydrates with potatoes, rice, and sugar-free chips or crackers. Read labels to make sure that there are no trans fats in any of these items. Sweet potatoes and baked potatoes are an excellent carbohydrate alternative to sugar. Most kids enjoy baked potatoes with olive oil just as much as butter and sour cream.

6. Read carefully the nutritional information on all of the staples in your pantry. Chicken stock, for example, may have added sugar.

7. You will find that many condiments have sugar added. Beware, for example, how much sugar and acidity is in ketchup. Condiments should be enjoyed in moderation, not with every meal.

Consider a diet that has healthy protein and good fats, including eggs, poultry, fish, avocado, olive oil, wild or brown rice, tofu, vegetables, and salad greens. The goal is not to be unrealistic and try to eliminate all sugar entirely. Instead, our hope is that you are more aware that sugar is found in so many types of food and that breaking your child's (or your own) sugar addiction requires strong will, dedication, and knowledge.

Eating Lean, Clean, Green, and Alkaline

The list of foods we are not allowed to eat can feel endless and restrictive, but possibilities for healthy and delicious alternatives abound. Our guidelines for healthy eating for an anti-reflux family are simple: remember to eat lean, clean, green, and alkaline.

Lean. According to the USDA, in 2014, the average American consumed 181 pounds of meat a year; that's not lean and much of it isn't healthy.[107] (This is down from 200 pounds per capita a few years ago.) Try to limit your family's consumption of red meat to no more than once a week or less and chicken to once or twice a week at most. Both beef and chicken contain lots of cholesterol. Consider spending more on antibiotic-free and hormone-free meats.

In fact, most animal products including dairy, eggs, poultry, beef, and pork, have relatively high levels of trans fats and cholesterol that can cause obesity, diabetes, heart disease and some cancers. Your family does *not* need to have meat every day.

Clean. Avoid buying foods with ingredients and additives you can't pronounce—better yet, look up unfamiliar ingredients on your smart phone! Remember that the point of processing food is to enable the food to sustain a longer shelf life. Most likely, added acid and other chemicals are what is allowing that extended expiration date. Cured meats and cold cuts contain unhealthy preservatives like nitrites, sodium, acids, and worse.

We all tend to buy the same types of foods week after week, so start reading nutrition labels and break up your routine. For example, that energy bar that you love for a quick boost may be loaded with preservatives and sugar. Choose an organic option. Revamping your shopping habits is going to be hard at first. Bring your reading glasses, because often the ingredients are shown in tiny print.

Green. By green we mean good for the environment as well as eating a variety of plants. Whenever you can, buy organic. Not only is it healthier, restrictions on pesticides and other harmful practices are generally better for the planet. Again, begin looking at labels in the supermarket. Fortunately, many stores now have entire sections dedicated to organic foods. Don't forget about your local farmers' market, and buy local and what is in season.

There is no substitute for veggies and salads. Plan every dinner to include some greens. While organic fresh fruit is great, limit your family's consumption of acidic fruits like green apples and citrus. Less acidic fruit choices include bananas, red apples, and pears. Most kids love berries and melon. They're good choices even though they are somewhat acidic. Encourage children to mix fruit in bland non-sugary yogurt. If they need some added sweetness, a bit of organic raw honey can do the trick.

Alkaline. We know that a diet that is too acidic results in acid reflux. (For a refresher, turn back to "Why a Low-Acid (Alkaline) Diet Is Important for Refluxers," page 4). Avoiding acid means avoiding beverages in cans and bottles. Stay away from juices, sodas, lemonade, iced tea, energy drinks, and seltzer. Teach your children to drink water and to say "no thanks" to all the other options. By the way, beverages that are acidic often are loaded with sugar and/or unhealthy chemicals.

At the initial transition to a low-acid diet, you may want to try to have your children eat and drink only food and beverages that are above a pH of 5.0.[1-4] Try this for two weeks. You can apply this system to baby food as well. We realize this is not easy. Try your best. For the babies, we have provided a list of the pH of different baby foods as well as fresh fruit and vegetables on pages 29–30 and 202–205. Try to create your own shopping list for less acidic choices. In general, just remember, the higher the pH (the less acidic), the better.

Exercise and Your Child

With diet and lifestyle being the biggest influencers on health, we would be remiss if we spoke only of nutrition and not of exercise. When we say exercise, we mean to get moving. It is not necessary to ask your kids to pack a gym bag on a daily basis and have great expectations of ninety-minute cardio/weight training workouts. Who needs that pressure? You don't have to spend money on a gym membership, unless your child really wants one. Rather, talking to kids about being aware of when they've been sitting too long and encouraging them to get out and about at least thirty minutes a day will help them learn to stay mindful of their sedentary habits.

Just as it is important to teach children at the youngest age possible about healthy eating, the value of exercise should be instilled with equal vigor.

Toddlers should be spending most of their time without electronic devices and media. If possible, spend time with them outside and monitor daycare facilities' practices when it comes to what your child plays with and for how long.

For school-age children up to twelve, ask them what they do during recess. Since we can't be in school watching them, we don't know if our children are getting the activity that recess is supposed to provide. Talk with their physical education teachers about the curriculum and find out what activities your child is gravitating toward. We had a patient whose kids loved to wear an exercise tracker, which they could check all day long to gauge if they "got their steps in." They even had a healthy family competition, with rewards at the end of each week.

Again, kids (and adults) do not have to be doing "organized" activities in order to be exercising. Finding and nurturing children's natural interests are great first steps in helping them learn to love moving.

Teens are challenging in every way, especially when it comes to exercise. Unless they are already committed to a sport or other activity like dance or martial arts, it's difficult to teach children to exercise when it's late in the game. Exercise can include just about everything from doing chores, to climbing stairs, to parking on the other side of the parking lot

Just Because It Says "Organic" on the Label . . .

We respect each family's decision of whether buying organic is worth the extra expense. Regardless, we need to get one thing straight: organic is not synonymous with healthy. Just because the label says organic does not mean it is sugar-free, low in fat, or alkaline.

The reality is that in our capitalistic society, where success is measured by how much of a product is sold, marketing ploys abound. There is no proof that eating organic will prevent the diseases or symptoms that this book is concerned with. Daily conversations have taught us that nearly all parents naïvely believe with complete confidence that if a fruit juice and/or milk has a label stating that it's "organic," it must be "good" or healthy, in whatever quantity.

There is an immediate association that "organic" means "safe." Not true. Organic or not, the focus must be on reducing the consumption of sugary beverages in young children to a strict minimum. We can't overemphasize the critical importance of this fact as a tool for controlling acid reflux. If a food is in a package, it has been processed, and organic or otherwise, there is still a significant amount of acid lurking.

at the mall. Encouraging baby steps in teenagers can go a long way toward helping them set achievable exercise goals.

Sedentary parents raise sedentary kids, so perhaps it's time to shake up your family's routine for the sake of helping your children develop better habits. We all want our children to do better and have more than we do. Of course, that means we want them to be healthier than we are too!

Meal Planning

This is not the time to leave you high and dry. It's not only our mission to educate you on lifestyle choices that can help keep your family an anti-reflux family, we also want you to enjoy eating and meal planning. Please consider photocopying this one-week meal plan template for your refluxing child. And, in addition, you can even make a meal plan for yourself or for your whole family.

MEAL PLAN FOR_____

	MONDAY	TUESDAY	WEDNESDAY
BREAKFAST			
SNACK			
LUNCH			
SNACK			
DINNER			

THE WEEK OF _____

THURSDAY	FRIDAY	SATURDAY	SUNDAY

Reflux Trigger Foods

Some foods are known as reflux trigger foods. They may have adverse effects on the LES (lower esophageal sphincter) or even on the stomach itself. Unfortunately, because everyone is different, it is hard to generalize a treatment for reflux. Certain foods such as onions, garlic, or tomatoes may be a reflux trigger for one person, but not for another. Keeping a food diary may help you identify your child's trigger foods. Once she reaches an appropriate age, ask your child to take notice of whether she has more upper airway symptoms after eating certain foods. Here's a list of the most commonly known reflux trigger foods (with the most common and notorious listed first):

- Chocolate
- High-fat meat
- Deep-fried food
- Alcohol
- Green apples
- Onions
- Garlic
- Nuts
- Bell peppers (green are worse than red)
- Cracked pepper
- Tomatoes
- Processed meat
- Cow's milk
- Cheese
- Coffee
- Bread (especially if you or your child is gluten-sensitive)

School Lunch: Problems and Solutions

Young children are very active and have high metabolisms so parents and caretakers often give preschoolers mid-morning and afternoon snacks.

Fresh fruits including ripened peaches, grapes cut into halves or quarters, red apple slices, pieces of melon, and bananas are best go-to options. If your child goes to daycare or school, be sure to review the monthly menu so that you know what your child is eating for both meals and snacks. Many preschools and daycares are now following best practice guidelines and serving only water and milk and are "no juice" programs. If your school is feeding your toddler canned meats and pasta or any other processed items, your child is likely taking in too much acid and may be at increased risk for acid reflux.

Many parents tell us that they pack and provide all foods and beverages needed for their child at daycare. When we review the contents of these packed lunches, common items include squeezable yogurt tubes, pouches of fruit purees, pouched sugary drinks, applesauce, puddings, and fruit cups in syrup. This is simply too much sugar. These items are also frequently high in acidity.

After many years of reflecting on our own behavior as parents, it makes complete sense that cutely packaged, conveniently compact, and comparatively non-perishable pre-processed items appear at first glance to be great choices. The food industry knows and counts on parents choosing convenience over nutrition, especially when it's so difficult to determine what is truly "healthy." When an item is labeled "Organic," "For Babies," "For Kids," and/or "100% Natural," it's got to be healthy, right? Unfortunately, we can't trust products based on how they are labeled. The more non-perishable an item is, whether on the shelves or in the refrigerated section of grocery stores, the more it is likely to have been acidified in order to prevent spoiling. The continued prevalence of acid reflux in toddlers and school-age children is due, in large, to a lack of awareness, which leads to uninformed shopping and unhealthy meal planning.

Let's return to options for packing for a healthy day at daycare: If you are able to cook at night for dinner, leftovers are a great choice. Dr. Julie recalls growing up in Taiwan during her elementary school years. Every night after dinner, her mother packed the next day's lunch in a metal rectangular box. It would often include a balanced variety of rice, meat or fish, vegetables, egg, and at times, a thermos of a broth-based soup of some kind.

Each of her fellow students came to school carrying similar metal lunch boxes, tied with butcher's twine and labeled with metallic "dog tags." As they walked into the classroom, the children dropped off their lunches into a large crate, which was transported to a steam room to be reheated. At lunchtime, school children ate these hot lunches and no "sweets."

Healthy options for daycare and preschool lunches and snacks include fresh fruit like red apples, honeydew, grapes, and bananas (sliced or whole). Other options include grilled chicken breast (cut up into appropriately-sized chunks), fresh mozzarella, cheese slices (not necessarily cheese sticks, which are often difficult to digest), sweet potato chunks, peas, mashed potatoes, boiled pasta (with a little butter, salt, and parmesan), and boil-to-eat ravioli with a red sauce that does not have added sugar, and is made with whole tomatoes, and not tomato puree.

Often parents want to pack their child yogurt, because children love the creamy and sweet combination of most yogurt and yogurt products. Choose yogurts with as little sugar as possible, and add fresh fruit to sweeten. Little pouches of "fruit snacks" (gummy snacks) are another popular and problematic item for children. Unfortunately, the word "fruit" misleads many parents to believe these sugary treats are healthy. Fruit snacks are essentially gummy candy packed with sugar. Remember, children, like adults, love something crunchy. Crackers and healthy chips that contain natural ingredients make for a satiating treat to include with lunch.

For elementary school-aged children, lunch can be a challenge. When asked, most tell us that for lunch they eat what is provided by the school—usually pizza, hot dogs, and chicken nuggets. Some schools do offer "healthy" options, but standards vary greatly from one public school to the next. All public schools provide milk for lunch as the beverage of choice but not just 2% white cow milk; strawberry and chocolate flavors are equally popular options.

Many children tell us that their school lunches are "disgusting." They even report skipping lunch all together, which explains a tendency to binge on items with excessive sugar and calories upon returning home from school. In this situation, packing a healthy lunch can be a welcome change for everyone.

Most homemade lunches typically include a sandwich, some type of chip or cracker, and, perhaps, a piece of fruit. As mentioned above, leftovers can be a great option unless they need re-heating. For variety, a Caesar salad makes for a tasty alternative; one can easily pack some cut grilled chicken breasts with romaine lettuce and a small amount of dressing. Cut fresh mozzarella squares with tomatoes, sprinkled with a drizzle of olive oil and freshly cut basil leaves, are another option. With a thermos, you can pack homemade chicken soup or leftover pasta. Break up the boring cold-cut sandwich routine!

Remember that on hot days, you may need to pack a small ice pack to ensure food safety. Until kids are able to peel and/or bite into whole fruit, cut fresh fruits into appropriate-sized chunks. Grains such as couscous, with the addition of some chopped vegetables and/or chicken, are a great option that can be enjoyed at room temperature. It's easy to prepare (the key is to season food so that it's not too bland).

The options of eating at school or packing a lunch should be part of a discussion you have with your child as you review the school menu together. Please talk to your child about what they are actually eating (or not eating) at school, and encourage drinking either water or white milk as opposed to flavored alternatives. Be sure to ask your older children if vendors sell fast foods on their campus, and, if so, discuss how often, if at all, your child should partake as a part of their daily school lunch.

Snack Options

Try matching a protein with whole grain or fruits and vegetables for optimal nutrition, such as:

Whole Grains	Protein	Fruits / Vegetables
Whole wheat crackers	Low-fat cheese	Apple or fresh fruit
Whole wheat bread	Peanut butter	Baby Carrots
Rice cakes	Hummus	Celery sticks
Whole corn tortilla chips	Roasted nuts	Salsa
Whole wheat tortilla	Turkey deli meat (not cured or smoked, nitrate free)	Raisins or dried fruit
Granola	Yogurt	Frozen blueberries

(Copyright; this table reprinted with permission from *A Healthier Wei*.[5])

How to Juggle Dinner with Soccer, Piano, Dance, Gymnastics, Swimming . . .

Previously we mentioned how the timing of when we eat can increase or decrease acid reflux. As most families have children involved in many activities or sports, your child is probably changing in the back seat of the car from one activity to the other while consuming intermittent slices of lukewarm pizza! The challenge for families is not only the logistics of "who is taking whom where," but the constant disruption of routine that makes a regular family dinner seem like an impossibility. Managing acid reflux is about the foods we eat and the time we eat them. Despite our maniacal schedules, we can beat the clock with healthy alternatives.

For preschool-aged children, we recommend that there be at least sixty to ninety minutes between dinner and bedtime, and for school-aged children about ninety minutes to two hours. Given that this is not feasible when practices and games end as late as 9:00 p.m., we encourage families to be aware and plan meal options that minimize risk of acid reflux. We try not to emphasize exact times but rather the point that as long as parents are thinking about their upcoming schedule and taking the time to make a plan, they are well on their way to a healthier lifestyle for their families. When there is no plan, oftentimes fast food on the way from one place to another will just have to do.

Try to make time for a brief Sunday night family meeting to review everyone's schedule for the week ahead. Ask questions like, "When are both parents home at the same time?" "Who has work obligations?" "Which child has what until when?" and "On which nights is it possible to have a sit-down family dinner?"

From the Case Files of Dr. Julie

A twelve-year-old, highly competitive gymnast had recurrent stomach upset and vomiting. She practiced twenty to twenty-five hours per week after school, usually from 5 p.m. to 8:30 pm. Since her mother was worried she wasn't getting sufficient calories, before practice she provided her daughter with a full dinner including items like lasagna and pasta with Alfredo sauce—really whatever the child wanted. Imagine doing tumbling runs, swinging on the bars, and doing summersaults with all that sloshing around in your belly! Gravity was simply working against her! We discussed foods and beverages to avoid in order to minimize acid reflux (processed sugar, sodas, highly fatty foods, and heavy cheese sauces like Alfredo). In this case, eating a lighter but high in protein meal as early before practice as possible, followed by a second light meal after practice (if necessary) provided a workable solution.

Many parents of athletes ask us what they should feed their child after school and before practices. This is an important question because depending on what your child eats, there can be high risk of acid reflux and delayed gastric emptying (the time it takes for stomach content to move out of stomach, into the small intestine). Here are key points for what to eat and when to eat relative to time of intense periods of exercise.[108]

- Eat high-carbohydrate meals and allow enough time for digestion prior to events.
- Limit high-fat protein such as peanut butter due to increased gastric emptying time.
- Learn about the glycemic index of foods. Eat high glycemic index foods during or after exercise and low-to-moderate index foods before exercise. High glycemic index foods include: potatoes, bagels, raisins, oatmeal, and sugar. Low-to-moderate index foods include: plain pasta, organic high protein bars, green beans, yogurt, and fruits such as apples and bananas.
- Avoid "sugar crash" by limiting high-glycemic, high-sugar items.
- Get adequate water and hydration all day, every day, and especially the day before competition.

Dining Out with Awareness

Most families probably eat out at the same places repeatedly and are familiar enough with the menu to identify the healthy and not-so-healthy menu items. How strictly you monitor your choices should be in direct proportion to how often your family dines out. If your family eats out nearly every night, making healthy choices is more critical. For families that eat out less often, maybe one night per week, larger portions, fried foods, and sugar-rich, gooey desserts high in fat may be enjoyed (but are likely to cause some acid reflux later that night). Human behavior and psychology may dictate a "splurge" mentality, rewarding good choices during the week with a one-night-a-week "cheat meal." Our suggestion is to encourage everyone to focus on making healthier choices at home, so you can indulge when you want to.

Those who plan ahead of time before going to restaurants end up making healthier choices and eat less than those who do not. True, you may be saying to yourself, "Who in the world has time to review the menu before showing up at the restaurant?" Let's keep it simple. Of course, adults will want an adult beverage with dinner, and children might complain if they don't get lemonade or a Sprite. It's okay. After a long week, we all want to enjoy a beverage in peace. While we suggest avoiding any soda intake, if you must order a soda, order half portions or split a single glass into two servings.

Always order a vegetable, whatever vegetable. Desserts in restaurants tend to be way over the top, so plan to order just one to share as family.

Try new foods when dining out. You may be surprised that your child may like sushi (maybe not the raw fish, but the rolls and cooked fish/seafood options, or vegetarian rolls like California rolls with imitation crab and avocado/cucumber). Most families love Chinese food. Order some soup as a way to curb appetite. Try to include stir fry vegetables with sauce on the side, instead of sweet and sour chicken or entrees where meats have been fried and then covered with sauces that are high in sugar and full of artificial coloring.

Here are some other ideas to minimize the damage done when eating out:

- Give children a choice between a sugary drink or dessert, but not both.
- Kids love Shirley Temples. Ask that they be made with club soda instead of ginger ale, in order to cut down on sugar. Plain water is better than carbonated water, but carbonated club soda is better than any soda, and with a splash of juice, the bubbles can seem "fancy" and make a special treat for children on special occasions.
- Bribe your kids with dessert by requesting they drink one or two glasses of water (depending on age and size) with their meal. They will be fuller and better hydrated.
- Ask for sweet potato fries instead of french fries.
- Go easy on condiments, and keep salt shakers away from the kids.
- Make sure no one is filling up on bread.
- Avoid the kid's menu (mostly fried junk foods), and order a few appetizers instead. There are likely some healthier choices like shrimp cocktail or salad. Order a variety of foods so that everyone is satisfied.
- Cleanse the palate. Once we get the taste of sugar, we naturally want more. After a meal and before dessert, offer a piece of parsley or a lemon

or orange slice to cleanse the palate of sugar. As a result, your child will likely eat less dessert. Ask for lemon slices, which typically can be added to water, so that everyone can break their sugar addiction!

- Be in the habit of not finishing everything on your plate; in fact, eat slowly, and ask around the table if everyone is getting full. Save half of an entrée for the next day, especially when dessert is going to be ordered.

Invite your children to be active participants in choosing restaurants and encourage discussions on why you are helping them moderate certain foods. Explain that dining out is an important opportunity to bring the family together and catch up on the day, not an excuse to overindulge and pig out. When children feel empowered and connected and not restrained and denied, they are encouraged to take more active roles in their health and learn tools and strategies that will benefit them well into their teenage years—where they'll need all the help that they can get!

If a family has a history of a bad diet, it's not so easy to get healthy unless everyone is willing to make changes. It may seem like schedules, habits, preferences, and the food industry all conspire to make you and your children sick. You can, however, change. We recognize that there is no such thing as an ideal diet and that none of these changes is easy. The purpose of this section is to offer the principles necessary to serve as a foundation for a healthy future.

Bedtime Snacks: Stop the Madness!

If you allow your toddler to develop what seems like an innocent routine of eating a bedtime snack, s/he will generally continue this habit for years to come. Read below some common parental rationalizations for continuing to encourage this destructive habit and our responses to each:

She didn't eat a good dinner. If we teach children that they can choose not to eat the dinner you have painstakingly prepared, but that they can, instead, receive a preferred snack later on, including at bedtime, they will have no reason to change this behavior. Children are quite smart. Why would they work at trying new foods when they can dictate a diet of wonderful sugary treats!

Without a snack, my child won't go to sleep. Not true. It is true that during the newborn period, including the first twelve months of life, it is important that they receive enough calories to grow properly. This will mean feeding them day and night, even overnight when they wake up. After twelve months of age, if they haven't been taught how to fall asleep on their own while lying in the crib awake, parents should start teaching toddlers this skill. No child this age needs to be "rocked" or fed before bedtime so that they can go to sleep. Unless your child has medical reasons for why s/he must have food right before bed, all preschool-age children can be taught a routine that does not involve eating or drinking anything other than water for at least one to one-and-a-half hours before bedtime. When human bodies are sleeping, all systems are "down," and our digestive tract slows so that it may take even longer for us to digest foods or liquids. The secret that few parents or even doctors know is that children will actually sleep better without reflux or partially digested food stuff coming back up during sleep, which can cause cough, stuffy nose, and even the need to wake up and swallow their backwash.

He won't sleep well or sleep all night if he is hungry. As long as your child eats a good dinner, he should be fine until the morning. Worst-case scenario, your child goes to bed slightly hungry at night, and hopefully is encouraged to eat a great big breakfast the following morning. Sleep training is so important and so very difficult at this age. Talk to your pediatrician and search the Internet for books on this topic. Parents always want to come up with an explanation for why their non-speaking toddlers are waking up at night, and often we convince ourselves that hunger is the issue. When was the last time you woke up in the middle of the night because you were hungry? Biologically, humans and other animals do not need to eat while sleeping. Otherwise, they would constantly have to disturb their sleep in order to graze and hunt for prey!

My child is skinny, so the doctor said to give as much as she wants, whenever she wants. Always check with your child's doctor to make sure your child is not so skinny that they are diagnosed with "failure to thrive." If your child is healthy and growing appropriately in height, there is no absolute "percentage" that your child must reach for weight. Just because your child is not overweight or obese, does not mean you should let your child eat whatever s/he wants, whenever s/he wants. Remember that on the inside, your child may have high cholesterol and other lipid panel abnormalities like high triglycerides that may develop into medical diseases at some point in the future.

My child doesn't eat much at mealtime, so I give him snacks, as much as he asks. No parent wants to deny their child food. It just feels wrong and mean, and, frankly, snacks seem so benign. Cookies, crackers, fruit snacks . . . what's the big deal? Once again, if you want your child to eat better at mealtime, keep snacking limited to just one morning and one afternoon snack (after their morning and afternoon naps, respectively, to minimize chance of reflux).

Remember above all to eat lean, clean, green, and alkaline and try to limit sugar intake. Please see also Recommended Books, References, Web Links, and Community Resources, pages 206–209.

PART II

RECIPES FOR REFLUX REPAIR

Recipe List

Breakfasts

Soups

Salads

Side Dishes

Entrées

Snacks and Hors d'oeuvres

Desserts

Some of the recipes in this book are reproduced from Dr. Koufman's other books with the permission of copyright owners, The Reflux Cookbooks LLC, Katalitix Media LLC, and Dr. Jamie Koufman.

BREAKFASTS

Banana Ginger Energy Smoothie

Makes 3 one-cup servings | 180 calories per serving
Gluten-Free, Vegetarian, and Dairy-Free (depending on type of milk and yogurt used)

2 bananas, ripe
½ cup ice
2 cups milk (or almond milk)
1 cup yogurt
½ tsp fresh ginger, peeled and grated fine
2 tbsp brown sugar or honey (optional)

In a blender, add the ice, milk, yogurt, bananas, and ginger.

Blend until smooth.

Add sugar as needed.

Notes: • You can use cow's milk (1% recommended), Lactaid (lactose-free) fat-free milk, almond milk, or even soy milk. • Almond milk can be used for almost all of our recipes that have "milk" as an ingredient. • If you don't like ginger or you have none, substitute ¼ tsp orange zest, vanilla, or almond extract.

Roasted Beet & Blueberry Smoothie

Makes 4 servings | 70 calories per serving
Vegetarian, Gluten-Free, Dairy-Free

1–2 whole roasted beets
1–2 cups of fresh or frozen blueberries
2 cups unsweetened almond milk
½ cup of ice

Place all into a blender/mixer, blend until smooth.

Notes: • You can purchase beets already completely cooked and throw one or two in your smoothie to save time. • The beets add great color to this smoothie. • You can always add a banana to this or any other smoothie for pH-balancing, because as fruits go, banana is quite alkaline.

Green Smoothie

Makes 4 servings | 60 calories per serving
Vegetarian, Gluten-Free, Dairy-Free

2 cups of honeydew chunks
1 cup of spinach
½ cup green grapes
1 cup water
½ cup ice

Place all into a blender/mixer, blend until smooth.

Notes: • You can purchase melon already in chunks, but it is relatively expensive.
• When you prepare your melon, put the extra in the freezer for the future.

Berry Smoothie

Makes 4 servings | 65 calories per serving
Vegetarian, Gluten-Free, Dairy-Free

1 lb. of fresh strawberries—hulled and cleaned (may use frozen strawberries)
1 cup of raspberries
½ cup ice
1 cup unsweetened almond milk

Place all into blender/mixer, blend until smooth.

Notes: • You can always use alkaline water in smoothies or alkaline water ice cubes; this helps with pH-balancing, especially when other ingredients are acidic (such as berries). • To give creaminess to this smoothie, you can add 1 cup of low-fat frozen yogurt, which adds an additional 165 calories and dairy.

Berry Banana Smoothie

Makes 2 one-cup servings | 150 calories per serving
Vegetarian, Gluten-Free, Dairy-Free

2 ripe bananas
1 cup fresh or frozen berries
½ cup water
½ cup crushed ice

Add ingredients to blender, and blend till smooth.

Notes: • Bananas are alkaline and berries somewhat acidic, so this is a pH-balanced smoothie. • If you want, you can use alkaline water to make this smoothie almost pH-perfect. • Again, you can freeze alkaline water in ice trays for use in subsequent smoothies. • Frozen berries (especially cherries) are available in the frozen fruit section of your grocery, and a few can be added to almost any smoothie to add sweetness and rich color.

A Very Peachy Smoothie

Makes 2 one-cup servings | 190 calories per serving
Vegetarian, Gluten-Free, Dairy-Free

2 bananas
2 ripe peaches
½ cup water
½ cup crushed ice

Add ingredients to blender, and blend until smooth.

Notes: • As an option, you can add ¼ tsp cinnamon or replace peaches with pears, red apples, or a combination. • Again, if you prefer, you can almost always use almond milk instead of water in your smoothies.

Pear and Melon Smoothie

Makes 2 one-cup servings | 140 calories per serving
Vegetarian, Gluten-Free, Dairy-Free

1 banana
1 pear
1 cup fresh cantaloupe or honeydew melon
½ cup of crushed ice

Add ingredients to blender, and blend until smooth.

Notes: For smoothness, consider adding a two-inch piece of a peeled aloe vera leaf (the inside part). This addition is good for all smoothies. • Please do not use bottled or prepared aloe vera, just the fresh leaf that can be found in the vegetable aisle of most grocery stores.

Everyday Lox Omelet

Makes 1 serving | 175 calories per serving
Gluten-Free, Dairy-Free

3 eggs
2 slices of Nova Scotia smoked salmon (lox)
Canola cooking oil spray

Cut the smoked salmon into small pieces.

Crack 3 eggs into a small bowl, discarding two of the yolks, and lightly whisk with a fork.

Heat up frying pan over medium-high heat.

Spray with canola cooking spray, and add the eggs.

Cook eggs until almost done, and then flip with a spatula.

Place the lox on the omelet, then fold.

Cook 1 more minute, and serve.

Notes: This is a staple breakfast item that is easy to cook yourself or order out. • It doesn't get much simpler than, "I'll have a three-egg omelet with one yolk and lox." • Try to avoid using farmed fish; wild-caught is recommended.

Egg White Wrap with Dill or Basil

Makes 2 servings | 270 calories per serving
Dairy-Free

6 egg whites
2 tbsp chopped dill or basil
¼ tsp salt
1 tbsp olive oil
2 flour tortillas

Beat egg white with fresh dill or basil and salt. Heat oil in small pan on medium-high heat.

Scramble egg mixture until cooked through.

The tortilla needs to be heated in a skillet for 30 seconds to soften and flavor.

Place egg mixture on tortilla and roll.

Notes: • Use dill or basil, not both. • If you like, you could also add smoked salmon (lox) with the dill and tomatoes with the basil for a nonvegetarian option.

Healthy Good Morning Oatmeal

Makes 2 servings | 245 calories per serving
Vegetarian, Gluten-Free, Dairy-Free

1 cup water
1 cup soy milk (almond milk works
  well, too)
Dash salt

1 cup rolled oats
2 tbsp maple syrup
½ tsp vanilla extract

In a saucepan, heat up water and soy milk with salt.

Add oats.

Bring to a boil. Lower heat and cook 10 minutes, stirring regularly.

Add vanilla extract after oats have cooked.

Notes: • Fresh fruit—sliced bananas and berries or whatever—may be added after the oatmeal is cooked. • During the winter, you may want to use dried fruit, such as raisins or apricots.

OMG (Oh My Gosh) Pancakes

Serves 4 | 220 calories per serving

2 tbsp light brown sugar
½ cup oat flour
½ cup all-purpose flour
1 tsp baking powder
½ tsp nutmeg
2 large eggs
3 bananas, blended or food
   processed

2 tbsp (1 oz.) nonfat sour cream or
   buttermilk
Milk (to consistency)
1 tbsp butter (for cooking)
Maple syrup, as desired

Mix first six ingredients together in bowl.

Whisk in the sour cream or buttermilk, the eggs, and the bananas.

If the mixture is too thick, add milk a few tablespoons at a time.

Preheat a nonstick pan over low to medium heat. Wipe a paper towel that has been rubbed with butter on the bottom of the pan. (Remove the excess butter with the same paper towel, and use again before cooking the next pancake.)

Using a ladle, pour some batter into the pan.

Flip pancake when the underside is golden brown, and cook until no longer wet inside.

Keep warm until all the pancakes are ready.

Serve with maple syrup; can be topped with diced apples.

Notes: • Cooking in a nonstick pan allows you to use butter sparingly. • If you make the batter the night before, don't add the baking powder until just before cooking. • Also, adding a bit of finely diced fruit to the batter just before cooking gives these pancakes extra flavor and texture.

Buckwheat Waffles

Makes 4 servings | 165 calories per serving
Vegetarian, Dairy-Free

DRY MIX
½ cup buckwheat flour
½ cup white flour
1 tbsp palm sugar
¼ tsp baking soda
⅓ tsp baking powder

WET MIX
1 tsp vanilla extract
1 tbsp grape seed oil
1 cup soy milk (only use soy milk made of 2 ingredients: organic soybeans and water). Any additives (sugars, gums, stabilizers), will simply destroy the healthy result you are seeking.

In one bowl, whisk together the dry mix.

In another bowl, whisk together the wet mix.

Add wet to dry, stir gently, leaving lumps.

Add ¾ cup of mix to a waffle maker, and cook until done.

Notes: • *This is an outstanding breakfast dish with the wonderful flavor of buckwheat.*
• *Serve with some fresh fruit and a bit of maple syrup for a nice, sweet breakfast or brunch.*

Gluten-Free Pumpkin Banana Muffins

Makes 12 muffins | 130 calories per muffin
Vegetarian, Gluten-Free, Dairy-Free

⅓ cup quinoa flour
½ cup quinoa flakes
1 tsp baking soda
2 tsp baking powder
1 tsp cinnamon
½ tsp ground ginger
¼ tsp ground cloves

½ tsp salt
4 tbsp honey
2 eggs
2 very ripe bananas
1½ cup pumpkin puree (from can)
PAM cooking spray (or grape seed oil)

Preheat oven to 400°F.

In one bowl, whisk together quinoa flour, quinoa flakes, baking soda, baking powder, cinnamon, ginger, ground cloves, and salt.

In another bowl, whisk together honey, eggs, ripe bananas, and pumpkin puree.

Add contents of both bowls together; stir gently.

Spray muffin tins with PAM, or grease lightly with grape seed oil.

Divide the mixture in 12 small muffin tins, and bake at 400°F for 20–25 minutes.

Notes: • This, a gluten-free muffin, was the number one most requested new recipe from Dr. Jamie's readers. • The overall taste of this muffin is like pumpkin pie and will make your kitchen smell like Thanksgiving. • Be careful not to under- or overcook. You can use the old toothpick method to see if the muffins are done: stick a toothpick into a muffin and if it comes out "dry," without muffin mix on it, they are done. • We recommend a 12-muffin tin, because this makes relatively small muffins, and these muffins cook best when not too large. For this reason, a serving for breakfast may be two muffins.

SOUPS

Perfect Pea Soup

Serves 6 | 300 calories per serving

1 lb. split peas (soaked in cold water overnight)

2 qts. chicken stock

2 oz. (4 slices) thin-sliced prosciutto (fat removed, cut into small strips)

3 sprigs thyme

2 bay leaves

1 tsp salt (or more, as needed)

2 tbsp nonfat sour cream

3 slices white bread (crust removed, cut into ¼-inch pieces)

In a medium saucepan, place the drained peas, prosciutto, and chicken stock. Bring to a simmer.

Wrap the thyme and bay leaves with butcher's twine, and attach to the handle of the pot for easy removal. Cook for about 45 minutes.

Remove the thyme and bay leaves.

Use a hand blender, regular blender, or food mill to blend the soup to a silky-smooth texture.

Add salt to taste. (Normally very little is needed because the prosciutto is quite salty.)

Serve or cool for later use.

Preheat oven to 325°F. Place the cubes of bread (croutons) on a cookie sheet, and put in the oven until golden brown. Keep at room temperature until needed.

TO SERVE

Reheat the soup, stirring frequently with a wooden spoon.

Adjust consistency with chicken stock, as needed.

Serve in a soup bowl, garnished with the croutons and 1 tsp nonfat sour cream.

Notes: • If you don't have time to soak the split peas, blanching them in hot water will work as well. Do not add salt to the peas yet, as it interferes with the softening of the peas and slows down the cooking process. (The same applies to all beans.) • If you do not cook the split peas on a low simmer, the soup may burn on the bottom of the pot. • Cook the croutons in a very low-temperature oven (300° F) to lower the risk of burning them. • The soup tends to thicken as it sits on the stove. Add chicken stock to adjust the consistency. • Caution: The soup can scorch easily during reheating because of its starchy consistency. • Because we first trim the fat from the prosciutto, there is almost no fat in this recipe.

Black Bean and Cilantro Soup

Serves 3 | 70 calories per serving
Gluten-Free

8 oz. canned black beans (drained and rinsed with clear water)
1 pint chicken (or vegetable) stock
½ cup fresh cilantro (washed, roots removed, and chopped with the stems)
Salt to taste
1 tsp nonfat sour cream (for garnish, optional)

In a medium saucepan, bring the chicken stock to a boil. Add the beans, cilantro, and salt.

Cook 30 minutes on low heat.

Blend with a hand blender to the desired consistency.

Season as needed.

Serve in a soup bowl, and garnish with 1 tsp nonfat sour cream and a sprig of cilantro.

Notes: • The cilantro stems give the soup a bright, zesty flavor. • Add more chicken or vegetable stock if the soup is too thick.

Carrot and Potato Soup

Serves 4 | 65 calories per serving
Gluten-Free, Dairy-Free

1 lb. carrots (peeled, diced into
½-inch cubes)

12 oz. (2½ cups) Idaho potatoes
(peeled and diced into 1-inch cubes)

1 qt. chicken stock (vegetable stock
may be substituted)

1 tbsp fresh ginger (peeled and cut
into ¼-inch pieces)

1 tbsp fresh parsley (washed, stems
removed, cut into fine strips; dried
on a paper towel)

Place the carrots, potatoes, chicken stock, and ginger in a large saucepan. Simmer for about 40 minutes on low heat.

Place the soup into a blender and blend until smooth. Season as needed.

Serve in a bowl, and garnish with the parsley.

Notes: • If the soup becomes too thick, add more chicken stock. • This is a nice winter soup. • Instead of parsley, you can use cilantro.

Fresh Mushroom Soup

Serves 6 | 65 calories per serving

1 lb. domestic mushrooms
½ qt. whole milk
½ qt. chicken stock
2 bay leaves
3 sprigs thyme
Salt to taste
2 tsp Parmesan cheese, grated

4 sprigs flat-leaf parsley (stems removed, chopped fine, and dried in a paper towel)
2 slices white bread (optional: crusts removed)

Wash mushrooms 2–3 times by lifting them from a bowl filled with cold water. Proceed until the water is clear. (Mushrooms often have sand in them.)

Remove about ¼-inch from the bottom of the mushroom stem, cut in half lengthwise, and cut as thin as possible.

Place the milk, stock, thyme, and bay leaves in a saucepan and bring to a simmer. Add the mushrooms, and cook for about 40 minutes.

Remove the thyme and bay leaves. Using a high-speed blender, blend the soup to a smooth consistency.

Add salt to taste.

Place the soup into a bowl, and sprinkle with grated Parmesan cheese and chopped parsley.

Notes: • Do not use the water from the bowl after washing the mushrooms, as some of the dirt will reattach to the mushrooms. The best way to wash mushrooms is to have two bowls. Fill one with water, add the mushrooms, and agitate. Lift the mushrooms and place in the empty bowl. Then fill the second bowl with water and do the same until the mushrooms are clean. • Using a high-speed blender allows the soup to get velvety without adding any cream or fat. A hand blender will also work, but the consistency won't be as smooth. • If the soup is too thin, blend one or two slices of white bread (crust removed) with the finished soup. The starch from the bread will slightly thicken it. • If you like a deeper taste to the soup, you can add about 1 tbsp dried mushrooms. • You can also garnish the mushroom soup with sautéed sliced mushrooms that have been caramelized in a tablespoon of olive oil or butter. The caramelized (brown-colored) mushrooms add a great earthy taste.

Egg Drop Soup

Makes 4 servings | 130 calories per serving
Gluten-Free, Dairy-Free

4 cups chicken stock
¼ tsp salt
¼ tsp minced fresh ginger root (not bottled)
3 tbsp water

1½ tbsp corn starch
4 egg whites
Cilantro, chopped for garnish (optional)

Heat chicken stock on medium-high heat.

Add salt and ginger, and bring to a boil.

In a small bowl, stir in water and corn starch until smooth and set aside.

Separate the eggs, and whisk them in a small bowl, then set aside.

Drizzle egg a little at a time into the boiling broth while stirring.

Gradually stir in the corn starch until desired consistency.

Serve hot, topped with cilantro (optional).

Notes: • This soup makes a great start for any family meal. • This classic and traditional Chinese dish can be made vegetarian by using vegetable stock in place of chicken stock. • Addition of cilantro brightens this dish a lot.

Tuscan White Bean Soup

Makes 4 servings | 400 calories per serving
Vegetarian, Gluten-Free, Dairy-Free

¼ cup olive oil
1 stalk celery, diced
1 carrot, diced
1 cup fresh peas
2 tsp sea salt
2 bay leaves
1 tsp dried oregano
1 tsp dried thyme

½ tsp dried rosemary
¼ cup dry white wine
4 cups vegetable stock
1 can white beans, rinsed and drained
1 cup chopped basil
¼ cup parsley (Italian parsley preferred)

In a large soup pot, heat olive oil.

Add vegetables, salt, and spices, and cook 10 minutes.

Add white wine, and cook 5 minutes.

Add stock and beans.

Bring to simmer; season to taste.

Add basil and parsley.

Notes: • This is a classic Northern Italian soup. • To make this a one-pot meal: add 1 to 2 cups of cooked pasta. Bowties or orzo pasta are excellent. • For lunch, have this soup with a salad and a hearty bread if you are gluten eater.

Southern Black-Eyed Pea Soup

Makes 4 servings | 155 calories per serving
Vegetarian, Gluten-Free, Dairy-Free

1 cup black-eyed peas, soaked
  overnight or for at least 8 hours
1 tbsp olive oil
1 carrot, diced
1 stalk celery, diced
1 bunch collard greens, chopped

1 tsp dried thyme
1 tsp dried oregano
4 cups vegetable stock
½ tsp sea salt
2 tbsp balsamic vinegar
¼ cup chopped parsley

Drain and rinse the soaked black-eyed peas.

In a hot soup pot, add olive oil.

Add carrot, celery, and collards, and sauté 5 minutes.

Add thyme, oregano, drained black-eyed peas, and stock, and bring to boil.

Lower heat, cover, and simmer 25 minutes or until the black-eyed peas are soft.

Add salt, vinegar, and parsley.

Notes: • You may want to consider doubling this recipe and make a big pot of this soup. • Like most bean soups, this one tastes even better the second day as all the favors merge; this soup has a relatively long shelf-life.

Corn Chowder

Makes 4 servings | 195 calories per serving
Vegetarian, Gluten-Free, Dairy-Free

2 tbsp olive oil
2 tsp sea salt
2 ears corn, shucked
2 medium potatoes, ¼-inch diced
1 large carrot, ¼-inch diced
1 stalk celery, finely diced
1 cup fresh, shelled peas

4 cups seaweed stock
1 sprig rosemary
2 tbsp fresh parsley, chopped
¼ cup fresh basil, chopped
Smoked paprika to garnish

In a hot soup pot, add olive oil, sea salt, and all the vegetables. Sauté over medium heat for 10 minutes.

Add stock and rosemary sprig, and bring to boil; then let simmer 3 minutes or until vegetables are fully cooked.

Add parsley and basil. Adjust salt if needed.

Garnish with smoked paprika, basil, and parsley

Notes: • This soup is best in the late summer and fall when fresh corn is in season. • Add a green salad and some hearty bread for a delightful fall lunch.

Borscht

Makes 4 servings | 175 calories per serving
Vegetarian, Gluten-Free, Dairy-Free

2 lbs. purple beets (3 large beets),
    peeled and ½-inch chopped
1 tbsp grape seed oil
1 tsp sea salt
2 tbsp fresh dill

3 cups water
1-inch piece of fresh horseradish or 1
    teaspoon dried horseradish powder
2 tsp balsamic vinegar (optional)

Preheat oven to 425°F.

Peel and dice beets and place in roasting pan with oil and salt. Stir to coat well. Cover and roast at 425°F for 30 minutes.

Combine the roasted beets, dill, water, horseradish, and balsamic vinegar in a blender and puree.

Chill and serve very cold in summer or bring to simmer, and serve hot in the winter.

Notes: • Borscht is a classic soup with many variations found throughout areas inhabited by Ashkenazi Jews. • Ice-cold borscht is incredibly refreshing in the summer, whereas hot borscht is warm and filling in winter.

Cantaloupe Gazpacho

Makes 2 servings | 180 calories per serving
Vegetarian, Dairy-Free

1 lb. (2 cups) cantaloupe (skin removed, seeded; cut into 1-inch pieces)
3 tbsp brown sugar or agave sugar
2 tbsp port wine
Dusting of finely grated nutmeg

Mix the cantaloupe, sugar, and port. Place in the freezer for about 4 hours.

Blend in a blender.

Finish with a dusting of nutmeg.

Serve immediately in a shot glass or small cup

Notes: • This is a refreshing summer soup. If using as a dessert, add more ice when blending. • You can use honeydew for this recipe as well, but use white port instead so that the soup maintains a light yellow-green color.

SALADS

Tricolored Salad with Walnuts & Cranberries

Makes 4 servings | 150 calories per serving
Vegetarian, Gluten-Free, Dairy-Free

2 handfuls of arugula (about ½ a regular size container)
½ sliced radicchio (that is usually about ½ of a whole radicchio)
3 Belgian endives, sliced into 1-inch pieces, discarding the stems

4 radishes cut in thin slices
15–20 shelled walnuts
½ cup of dried cranberries
2 tbsp balsamic vinegar
⅓ cup of olive oil

Put the arugula, radicchio, and endives into your salad bowl (a large one is best), and mix by hand.

Add the sliced radishes with the walnuts and cranberries on top.

Refrigerate and place on table with the balsamic vinegar and olive oil nearby.

Add the vinegar and oil at the very last minute before serving.

Notes: • *This is an amazingly diverse-textured and robust salad for company or your family.* • *You may want to ask if any guest is allergic to nuts before adding them (before tossing) if you have guests for dinner.* • *You can substitute other fine lettuces for the arugula.*

Calm Carrot Salad

Makes 2 servings | 235 calories per serving
Vegetarian, Gluten-Free, Dairy-Free

1 lb. carrots (peeled, trimmed, and grated)
¼ lb. mesclun greens
2 tbsp raisins
2 tbsp orange juice

1 tsp dried oregano
2 tbsp brown sugar
2 tsp olive oil
¼ tsp salt

In a bowl, mix the raisins, orange juice, oregano, brown sugar, olive oil, and salt. Let sit for about 5 minutes.

Pour the dressing over the carrots, and mix thoroughly.

Season with additional salt, as needed.

Serve over a few mesclun leaves.

Notes: • The infusion of oregano into the orange juice brings out its flavor. • Even with some orange juice, this salad is not very acidic; it is pH-balanced.

Spinach and Arugula with Apples and Pears

Makes 3 servings | 85 calories per serving
Gluten-Free

2 cups spinach
1 cup arugula
3 tbsp orange juice
1 Golden Delicious or else any red apple (peeled and grated on a coarse grater)

1 pear (peeled and diced to ½-inch cubes)
1 tbsp Parmesan cheese, grated
1 tsp sesame seeds, toasted
Salt to taste

Pour the orange juice over the apples and pears to keep them from turning brown (it slows the oxidation process).

Wash the spinach and arugula several times until clean. One way is to use a salad spinner. Another is to plunge the greens into a large bowl filled with cold water, remove, and repeat as needed. Keep washing until you no longer see sand on the bottom of the bowl.

Dry thoroughly: a salad spinner is easiest.

Toast the sesame seeds in a pan on the stovetop or in the oven until golden brown. Transfer them to a bowl or plate immediately to avoid burning.

Mix the spinach, arugula, apple, pear, Parmesan cheese, orange juice, and salt.

Present on a plate, and sprinkle with sesame seeds.

Note: • This salad can be served with sesame sticks or toasted whole-wheat bread.

Kale Salad with Almonds and Apples

Makes 4 servings | 175 calories per serving
Vegetarian, Dairy-Free

Half a bag of organic kale (5 oz.),
finely chopped
¾ to 1 honey crisp apple, finely
diced
¼ cup of honey-roasted almond
slices

2 tsp of honey (to coat wooden
salad paddles); you can substitute
with pure maple syrup
1 tsp of fresh lemon juice
2 tbsp of extra virgin olive oil
2 tbsp of balsamic vinegar

Combine chopped kale and apple into a salad bowl. Drizzle with olive oil, lemon juice, and balsamic vinegar.

Drizzle honey on the salad paddles, then toss the kale and apples. Sprinkle almond slices if desired, then gently toss once or twice before serving.

Notes: • This salad is simple and nutritious with awesome crunch. • As an alternative to honey crisp apples, Fuji apples are great. • You can search YouTube for Julie Wei Kale Salad.

Spring Salad with Mission Figs

Makes 3 servings | 210 calories per serving

8 to 10 ripe Mission figs
6 to 8 oz. spring mix
8 cherry tomatoes (halved)

2 oz. goat cheese
Drizzle of honey
Balsamic glaze salad dressing

Cut off the stems and bottoms of figs, then cut each into halves.

Place the salad mix into bowl, then sprinkle tomatoes and figs on top.

Sprinkle with goat cheese.

Drizzle with balsamic dressing and a little bit of honey.

*Notes: • You can also add cubed fresh mozzarella or sprinkle almond slices if desired.
• The small amount of vinegar is okay for most people with reflux.*

Spanish Bean Salad

Makes 6 servings | 290 calories per serving
Vegetarian, Gluten-Free, Dairy-Free

¼ lb. green beans, cut in ½-inch
   lengths, blanched
1 can chickpeas
1 can kidney beans
1 can black-eyed peas
1 large carrot, grated
1 tsp dried rosemary
2 tsp dried oregano

1 tsp dried thyme
¼ cup chopped parsley
3 tbsp olive oil
3 tbsp sherry vinegar
2 tsp sea salt
1 tsp mustard powder
1 tbsp lemon zest
¼ cup fresh parsley, chopped

Blanch the green beans by dropping them in boiling water for 5 seconds. Rinse under cold water, and drain.

Rinse the 3 cans of beans well, and drain.

Place all ingredients in a large bowl, and mix well.

Let marinate 2 hours before serving

Notes: • The combination of the dried herbs, olive oil, and sherry vinegar create a very refreshing salad for all seasons. • Like all bean salads and soups, consider making this one a day ahead to allow the flavors to fully develop and blend.

Brussels Sprout Slaw

Makes 4 servings | 75 calories per serving
Vegetarian, Gluten-Free, Dairy-Free

20 Brussels sprouts, shredded
10 basil leaves, chopped
1½ tbsp sesame oil

1 tbsp rice vinegar
2 tsp mirin
1½ tbsp tamari (soy sauce)

Toss all ingredients in a bowl together, and let marinade ½ hour before serving.

Notes: • This is a Japanese variation on the classic slaw idea. • Regular cabbage and/or red cabbage can be used or a combination of both.

Roasted Portobello Mushroom Salad

Makes 4 servings | 115 calories per serving
Vegetarian, Gluten-Free, Dairy-Free

SALAD
2 portobello mushrooms, stem and gills removed
1 tbsp olive oil
¼ tsp sea salt
1 large bunch arugula, chopped
½ head radicchio, shredded

DRESSING

2 tbsp olive oil
2 tbsp balsamic vinegar
¼ tsp dried thyme
¼ tsp dried rosemary

¼ tsp dried oregano
¼ tsp dried sage
¼ cup fresh parsley
1 tsp sea salt

Trim, wash, and dry the mushrooms.

Brush the mushrooms on all sides with olive oil, and rub a little salt into them.

Place on a baking tray and roast at 400°F for 10 minutes. Then turn them over and roast another 10 minutes.

Slice mushrooms and arrange on top of a bed of arugula and radicchio.

In a separate bowl, whisk together salad dressing ingredients, and pour dressing over mushrooms and greens.

Notes: • Some very nice Italian flavors give the mushrooms a delicious taste, enhanced by the peppery arugula and the bitterness of radicchio. • The color contrast between the three main ingredients is quite striking on the plate.

Leafy Green Salad

Makes 4 servings | 132 calories per serving
Vegetarian, Gluten-Free, Dairy-Free

SALAD

4 cups torn salad greens mixture

1 cucumber, diced

1 carrot, grated

1 purple beet, grated

1 tbsp sesame seeds, toasted

10 olives, not oil cured, sliced

DRESSING

2 tbsp balsamic vinegar

2 tbsp olive oil

¼ tsp dried thyme

¼ tsp dried marjoram or oregano

½ tsp dried mustard powder

¼ tsp sea salt

Tear leaves by hand instead of by knife to prevent discoloring.

Whisk dressing ingredients in a bowl, and pour over salad greens, coating the dressing onto the leaves. Drain excess dressing.

Arrange other ingredients decoratively over the salad greens, and serve immediately.

Notes: • A very quick and easy everyday salad with a variety of colors, textures, and flavors. • This salad dressing is not too acidic and can be used for lots of different salads.

Wilted Kale Salad

Makes 4 servings | 115 calories per serving
Vegetarian, Gluten-Free, Dairy-Free

1 bunch kale, stalks removed, leaves chopped very small
1 tbsp balsamic vinegar
½ tsp sea salt
1 carrot, grated

1 tbsp grated lemon zest
1 tbsp pumpkin seeds
1 tsp mirin
1 tbsp olive oil

In a bowl, massage the balsamic vinegar and salt into the kale. Let sit for 30 minutes.

Add the rest of the ingredients, and blend well to coat the kale leaves.

Notes: • Kale has received tremendous popularity in recent years due to its versatility, nutritional value, and ease of cultivation. • This is an easy everyday, flavorful dish.

SIDE DISHES

Roasting Vegetables

You can roast just about anything, simply have oven heated to 400°–425°F, cut vegetables into similar-size pieces, toss in extra virgin olive oil (EVOO), and season with salt and pepper.

Experiment by sprinkling in other seasonings such as paprika, cumin, cinnamon, etc. Toss all vegetables on baking sheet using your hand until evenly coated, then roast for about 20–40 minutes, depending on the vegetable and how much is on your pan. If garlic or onions are trigger foods, then avoid those in your recipes. Note: With a few tweaks, every roasted vegetable recipe can be made vegetarian, gluten-free, and dairy-free. This is the case with many other recipes.

Roasted Cauliflower

Makes 4 servings | 96 calories per serving
Vegetarian, Gluten-Free

1 head of cauliflower
2 tbsp olive oil
½ tsp minced garlic (optional)

1 tsp garlic salt
½ tsp paprika
¼ tsp cumin (optional)

Preheat oven to 400°F.

Cut the cauliflower into florets. Either flip it upside down so that you are looking at the base and use a knife to carefully cut out the core, or cut the head in half, so you can see where the core is, and cut into florets.

Place florets onto a baking sheet and drizzle with olive oil and garlic. Then sprinkle seasoning, tossing evenly until the florets are covered by the oil and seasoning.

Place into oven, roast for 25 minutes, take out immediately and serve. You may use the leftovers in a salad.

Notes: • You can use curry powder, smoked paprika, sumac, or other seasonings to create different flavors. • Once roasted, you can add cauliflower to arugula with large white beans and shaved parmesan and make a great salad with olive oil and lemon juice as dressing; use only a few drops of lemon. • For those with garlic as a trigger food, you should know that garlic powder and garlic salt are less likely to trigger reflux than fresh garlic. Just the same, if you are sensitive to garlic, feel free to leave it out of any of our recipes.

Roasted Root Vegetables

Makes 6 servings | 100 calories per serving
Vegetarian, Gluten-Free, Dairy-Free

2 sweet potatoes (peeled and cut into 1½-inch chunks)
3 large carrots (peeled and cut into similar-size chunks)
1 small or ½ large red onion (cut into similar-size pieces)
½ tsp minced garlic

1 tsp salt (or 1 tsp garlic salt)
1 tsp pepper
Chopped curly or flat parsley to sprinkle on top when done (optional)
2 tbsp olive oil

Preheat oven to 400°F.

Mix all ingredients and place on baking dish. Use hands to mix evenly, then place into oven. Check at about 30 minutes. If some sides are golden brown, then it's likely done.

Notes: • You can experiment with different root vegetables, including turnip, taro, a variety of sweet onions, rutabaga, yams and potatoes. • Be sure to cut the vegetables all into similar sizes when roasting. • Combine a variety of colors for a beautiful side dish.

Roasted Asparagus

Makes 4 servings | 80 calories per serving
Vegetarian, Gluten-Free, Dairy-Free

1 lb. of asparagus
2 tbsp of olive oil
Salt and pepper

Preheat oven to 400°F.

Trim asparagus by cutting off the bottom inch where it's "woody" and pale.

Place entire spear across baking sheet or cut into ⅓- or ½- or 2-inch pieces.

Hand toss in olive oil, place across baking sheet, and roast for 10–12 minutes.

Notes: • *If you prefer, you can line up all the spears of asparagus in a single layer, and brush olive oil over the surface.* • *Keep asparagus fresh and crispy when you get home from grocery store by standing the entire bunch in a bowl of water; and for maximum crunch, use within two days.* • *You may serve with a cut up hard-boiled egg sprinkled over the asparagus.*

Roasted Butternut Squash

Makes 4 servings | 110 calories per serving
Vegetarian, Gluten-Free, Dairy-Free

1 whole squash (or buy precut chunks in the produce section)
2 tbsp olive oil
Minced garlic (optional)
Salt and pepper

Preheat oven to 400°F.

Place even sized chunks onto baking sheet, toss with olive oil, and season as you wish.

Roast for about 30–40 minutes or until tender.

Notes: • *Roasted butternut squash can be used as an ingredient in many recipes, including soups, risotto, and pasta.* • *If buying whole squash, be careful when cutting; trim the top and bottom off, peel with a good vegetable peeler, and then cut into chunks. The wider bottom part contains seeds; cut around the seeds and discard.*

Roasted Beets

Makes 4 servings | 55 calories per serving
Vegetarian, Gluten-Free, Dairy-Free

3 large red beets
1 tbsp olive oil
3 square sheets of aluminum foil (about 10-inches x 10-inches)

Preheat oven to 400°F.

Trim each beet by removing greens on top (you can sauté and enjoy leaves separately).

Trim bottom of each beet, and cut off the long hanging "root."

Trim across the top so it can stand when turned upside down.

Lay out each square of aluminum foil, and place each beet in center of foil.

Drizzle ½ tsp of olive oil over top and let it run down the beet.

Wrap the beet completely with the foil.

Place all 3 in a baking dish or pan.

Roast for 40–45 minutes (the larger the beet, the more time required).

Take out of the oven, and let cool.

Unwrap in kitchen sink, then run gently under water and use hands to peel. The skin should come off easily. Place in Tupperware for refrigeration for future use.

Notes: • Roasted beets make a great addition to any salad, couscous or smoothie. • To serve warm, cut into quarters or small cubes, and consider adding 2 tbsp of goat cheese crumbles with or without honey and salt and pepper to taste.

Roasted Sweet Potatoes

Makes 4 servings | 90 calories per serving
Vegetarian, Gluten-Free, Dairy-Free

4 whole sweet potatoes (large and relatively oval-shaped/symmetric in size/girth)

Preheat oven to 400°F.

Wrap each sweet potato completely in foil.

Place on baking dish and roast for one hour (ready when fork pierces easily through it).

Notes: • You may slit potatoes vertically into halves and enjoy as is, or remove foil and skin and serve on a plate cut up into chunks. You can even make mashed sweet potatoes. • Serve with small amount of butter or olive oil. You can sprinkle cinnamon powder and brown sugar, or salt and pepper.

Sautéed Green Beans

Makes 4 servings | 95 calories per serving
Vegetarian, Gluten-Free, Dairy-Free

1 lb. fresh green beans, trimmed on both ends and cut into half
1 tsp or 1 tbsp of minced garlic
2 tbsp olive oil

In a wok, or skillet (preferably not nonstick), heat oil on medium-high heat. Add minced garlic and trimmed green beans, and stir all around until all beans are coated with oil.

After 2–3 minutes, sprinkle water or 2 tbsp vegetable or chicken broth, and cover immediately so the "steam" can help cook the beans through. Keep covered for a about 2 minutes, uncover, stir until tender, about 10 minutes total.

Notes: • Add 2 tbsp of hoisin sauce to impart a fantastic Asian flavor to this dish.

Grilled Eggplant

Makes 4 servings, 65 calories per serving
Vegetarian, Gluten-Free, Dairy-Free

1 eggplant
1 tsp sea salt
1 tbsp olive oil

Slice eggplant ½-inch thick.

Sprinkle salt on eggplant slices and massage in gently.

Put eggplant in a colander to drain for 1 hour.

Brush eggplant slices with olive oil.

Roast at 425°F in single layer for 15 minutes. Then turn over and roast another 10 minutes or until eggplant is slightly charred.

Notes: • This is a favorite stand-alone side dish. • You can sprinkle the eggplant slices with dried spices such as rosemary and oregano or sumac.

Fennel Roasted Beets

Makes 4 servings | 60 calories per serving
Vegetarian, Gluten-Free, Dairy-Free

1 large purple beet, peeled, diced
1 small bulb fresh fennel, diced
1 tbsp grape seed oil
1 tsp sea salt
1 tsp balsamic vinegar (gluten-free is available)

Preheat oven to 425°F

Place peeled and diced beets and diced fennel in a roasting pan with oil and salt.

Cover and roast at 425°F for 30 minutes or until lightly browned and caramelized on the edges.

Toss with balsamic vinegar, and serve.

Notes: • This classic combination of fennel and beets is a favorite from Eastern Europe. • Fennel is very good for reflux and the combination of fennel and beets is uniquely flavorful!

Rice with Cumin and Turmeric

Makes 4 servings | 200 calories per serving
Vegetarian, Gluten-Free, Dairy-Free

1 cup jasmine rice
2 cups vegetable stock
1 tbsp olive oil

1 tsp sea salt
½ tsp cumin
½ tsp turmeric

Add all ingredients to a rice cooker; cook as rice cooker indicates.

Fluff the rice with a fork and serve immediately.

Notes: • If you don't have a rice cooker, you can use a regular pot with a lid. Using a regular pot, bring contents to a boil and then cover at low heat for 30 minutes. Then, turn off and let rest for at least ten minutes before fluffing and serving • If you are making more than a cup of rice, the correct proportion of liquid to rice is 3:2. • This dish has a beautiful golden color and goes great with almost everything, especially fish. • This rice is a versatile and popular platform for any and all stir-fry dishes or saucy main course recipes. • For an unusual and tasty breakfast, put rice in a bowl, add olive oil and microwave; then, top with a fried egg.

Roasted Mashed Root Vegetables

Makes 4 servings | 130 calories per serving
Vegetarian, Gluten-Free, Dairy-Free

2 small potatoes, peeled and cut into
1-inch cubes
1 large parsnip, peeled, cut into
1-inch cubes
1 medium sweet potato, peeled and
cut into 1-inch cubes

1 small celery root, peeled, cut into
1-inch cubes
1 tsp sea salt
1 tbsp grape seed oil
¼ cup fresh parsley, chopped

Preheat oven to 425°F.

Peel and roughly chop the root vegetables. Toss with oil and salt and place in a roasting pan; cover with foil.

Roast for 40 minutes or until slightly caramelized.

Mash the roasted root vegetables with a fork or masher.

Garnish with chopped parsley.

Notes: • If you love mashed potatoes, you will really love this dish as it is a glorified version, adding more flavors by using a variety of root vegetables. • Roasted cauliflower may also be added.

Taiwanese Dill with Ginger

Makes 4 servings | 100 calories per serving
Vegetarian, Gluten-Free, Dairy-Free

3 tbsp olive oil
2 slices of ginger
1 bunch of dill (about 3 to 4 cups)

1 tbsp rice wine
¼ cup water or vegetable stock
Salt to taste

Heat oil on medium-high heat, add ginger and sauté until fragrant, about 1 minute.

Add dill, rice wine, water, and salt to taste for 2 to 3 minutes. Serve hot.

Note: • Although dill is usually an herb, in this case it's used as a vegetable.

Roasted Butternut Squash Puree

Makes 4 servings | 90 calories per serving
Vegetarian, Gluten-Free, Dairy-Free

1 butternut squash, peeled, seeded, and diced
1 tbsp grape seed oil
1 tsp sea salt

Preheat oven to 425°F.

Combine the squash, grape seed oil, and salt in a roasting pan, and mix until the squash is well coated with both.

Cover with foil and roast for 30 minutes.

Puree with a fork, masher, or food processor.

Notes: • This Native American ingredient is packed with flavor and nutrition and can be used in so many recipes, from soups to desserts. • For a variation to this recipe, add ½ tsp cinnamon to the puree. • You can also try adding chopped dried fruit and chopped pistachios.

Roasted Asparagus with Black Olives

Makes 4 servings | 155 calories per serving
Vegetarian, Gluten-Free, Dairy-Free

1 lb. asparagus, trim 2 inches off the bottom
¼ cup black olives, pitted, chopped
2 tbsp chopped parsley
2 tbsp white wine
1 tbsp olive oil

Preheat oven to 425°F.

Combine all ingredients in a bowl, and mix well.

Place on a baking sheet in a single layer, and roast uncovered 15 minutes or until asparagus is tender.

Notes: • When asparagus starts to come into season, this remarkable vegetable should make many appearances in your kitchen. • This is an easily prepared Italian spring side dish.

Anadama Bread

Makes 2 loaves | 95 calories per serving
Vegetarian, Dairy-Free

1 cup soy milk
1 cup water
2 tbsp blackstrap molasses
1 tsp dried yeast

2 tsp sea salt
2 cups cornmeal
2 cups white flour

Add yeast and blackstrap molasses to warm water (100°F), and whisk.

Let sit 5 minutes until foamy.

Add soy milk, sea salt, and whisk.

Slowly start to incorporate flour and cornmeal into the yeast mixture. Begin at first with a spoon. Place the dough on a flat surface, and knead with your hands for 10 minutes until smooth and shiny. Add more flour if it gets too sticky.

Brush dough with olive oil, place in bowl, cover with a towel, and let sit about one hour or until dough has doubled in size.

Cut dough in half, shape into loaves, cover, and let rise another hour or until doubled in size.

Bake in preheated 500°F oven for 25 minutes.

Notes: • *Traditionally made with cow's milk, this vegan version uses soy milk; if you prefer, you can substitute almond milk or 2% cow's milk—your choice.* • *The combination of corn and wheat provides wonderful flavor and texture, slightly sweetened and darkened by the molasses.*

Rustic Whole Wheat Bread

Makes 2 loaves | 100 calories per serving
Vegetarian, Dairy-Free

2 cups water
1 tsp dried yeast
1 tbsp agave
2 tsp sea salt

2 cups white flour
2 cups whole wheat flour
1 tbsp olive oil

Add yeast and agave to warm water (100°F) and whisk.

Let sit 5 minutes until foamy.

Add sea salt and whisk.

Slowly start to incorporate flours into the yeast mixture. Begin at first with a spoon. Place the dough on a flat surface, and knead with your hands for 10 minutes until smooth and shiny. Add more flour if it gets too sticky.

Brush dough with olive oil, place in bowl, cover with a towel, and let sit about one hour or until dough has doubled in size.

Cut dough in half, shape into loaves, cover, and let rise another hour or until doubled in size.

Bake in preheated 500°F oven for 25 minutes.

Notes: • If you have never baked bread before, this is a good basic recipe to start with. • Please look at videos online to learn the basics of kneading and rising. • Baking bread is a very meditative practice for many people, including those who do not otherwise cook.

Emperor's Jade Fried Rice

Makes 4 servings | 425 calories per serving
Vegetarian, Dairy-Free

4 tbsp olive oil
2 cups chopped spinach
2 cups chopped mustard greens
3 egg whites

1 egg yolk (optional)
4 cups of cooked rice
¼ cup of ¼-inch diced smoked tofu
Salt to taste

Heat 2 tbsp oil on medium-high heat, then add spinach, mustard greens, and sauté until wilted. Remove from heat, and drain excess water from pan.

Remove greens from pan and set aside.

Heat 2 tbsp oil on medium-high, whisk egg white and egg yolk, then add to the pan.

Scramble the eggs until cooked through.

Add rice, spinach/mustard greens mixture and smoked tofu, and mix well.

Season with salt.

Notes: • This is a great way to use up leftover rice: In fact, day-old rice works much better in any fried rice recipe. • This dish is usually made with other leftover ingredients as well, an everything-but-the-kitchen-sink approach.

ENTRÉES

How to Stir-Fry Anything & Everything

Makes 6–8 servings | 100–250 calories per serving (depending on ingredients)
Vegetarian, Gluten-Free, Dairy-Free

The authors stir-fry meals often. Of all of the recipes we offer, this can have thousands of permutations, using all different ingredients. If you don't have one, we recommend that you purchase an extra large, nonstick fry pan or wok. For all stir-frying, nonstick coating and olive oil in the bottom is the first step to stir-frying. Incidentally, never cook for just one meal because leftovers are great reheated, for omelets and for side dishes. The recipe below is Dr. Jamie's. Again, you can substitute any and all ingredients! Finally, all stir-fry dishes can be served on pasta, rice or as a side dish.

1–2 tbsp of ginger root, peeled and finely chopped

2 sweet Vidalia onions, coarsely chopped

2–3 handfuls of green beans cut into bite-size pieces

1–3 packages of sliced mushrooms (optional)

1 red bell pepper, de-seeded and cut into ½-inch pieces (optional)

1 small eggplant, skin partially removed so it is easy to cut into 1-inch cubes

1 package of extra-firm tofu cut into ½-inch cubes (optional)

1 pre-roasted cauliflower (cut into small bite-size florets)

1 tsp salt

1–2 tsp of soy sauce (recommended is Tamari, gluten-free soy sauce that is readily available in almost every grocery store). (Soy sauce is also optional.)

Nonstick pan spray

4–8 tbsp olive oil

Bring heat to high.

Spray pan or wok with nonstick spray and add 4 tbsp of olive oil.

Add the onions, mushrooms, green beans, bell pepper, and salt, and cook on high heat for 10–15 minutes.

Add other ingredients except for the already-cooked cauliflower and (optional) soy sauce and cook another 10 minutes, stirring often.

Add additional olive oil as needed to coat vegetables and to prevent any burning.

Last add cauliflower and soy sauce; reduce heat to medium.

When all of the veggies are cooked and the onions are caramelized, the dish is ready to eat.

Plate the rice or pasta and spoon the stir-fry on top.

Notes: • *Don't forget to time the cooking of your rice or pasta so that it is done before you are ready to dish the stir-fry.* • *Sweet Vidalia onions well-cooked, caramelized (clear and brown), are the least likely onions to cause reflux. You know they are real sweet Vidalias because you won't cry when you cut them up.* • *The longest-to-cook-through vegetables are added first; that is, the ginger, onions, green beans, mushrooms and red bell pepper.* • *Every ingredient is optional: you can use peanut or safflower oil for the cooking; other vegetable options that can be used include zucchini, squash, fennel, potato (small pieces), and virtually every vegetable. (We do not recommend tomato as it changes the texture of the stir-fry to mushy.)* • *To roast a cauliflower, cut out the stem and make the bottom flat so that it stands up in a roasting pan; put olive oil on the top and roast at 425° F for 35–45 minutes.* • *Instead, or in addition to ginger, you can use chopped 2–4 cloves of garlic.* • *Serve your stir-fry on rice (wild, white, black Japonica, or a combination) or your favorite pasta. (If wheat pasta is used, this is not a gluten-free dish.) Today, chickpea and brown-rice pastas are wonderful high-protein alternatives.* • *Best also served with a salad.* • *Get so you know your stove and vegetables so you get the best results; a hot gas stove cooks faster than an electric one.* • *The rice recipe on page 132 goes well with any stir-fry.*

Roasted Chicken

Makes 4 servings | 300 calories per serving
Gluten-Free, Dairy-Free

1 whole chicken, about 2 lbs. (yields about 3 cups of cooked diced chicken)
Salt and black pepper to taste
2 tbsp olive oil to rub the chicken

Preheat the oven to 350°F.

Place the chicken in a baking pan, rub with olive oil, and season with salt/pepper.

Bake uncovered for 1 hour, check the temperature to be sure it is at least 180°.

Take out the chicken and cover it, letting it cool at room temperature for about 30 minutes.

Remove bone. May serve with rice and vegetables, or shred diced chicken meat and use in soups, salads, grains such as couscous or quinoa, and sandwiches, etc.

Notes: • *You can add lemon or orange halves into the body cavity, along with onion and/or fresh herbs like rosemary for flavors.* • *Also, you can roast two chickens at the same time, and serve later in the week.*

Baked Salmon

Makes 4 servings | 220 calories per serving
Gluten-Free, Dairy-Free

4 salmon filets (4 oz. each)
2 tbsp olive oil
Salt and pepper to taste

Preheat the oven to 400°F.

Place the salmon in a baking pan and sprinkle with olive oil and minimal salt/pepper to taste.

Place in the oven with the skin side down and cook for about 12–15 minutes.

Notes: • Serve with plain rice and a green veggie, such as boiled/sautéed broccoli or green beans. • A little piece of left-over salmon is great in an omelet the next morning.

Broiled Salmon with Lemon

Makes 4 servings | 165 calories per serving
Gluten-Free, Dairy-Free

4 salmon filets (4 oz. each)
1 lemon, sliced into ⅛-inch thick round slices
Salt and pepper to taste

Preheat the oven to "broil."

Place the salmon filets on a baking sheet or in a pan, and cover entire surface with lemon slices.

Place in the oven and broil for 12–15 minutes or until lemon slices are "charred" and salmon is cooked through.

Note: • Serve with any sautéed vegetables or with salad.

Soy Miso Glazed Salmon

Makes 4 servings | 280 calories per serving
Gluten-Free, Dairy-Free

4 salmon filets (4 oz. each)
¼ cup soy sauce (regular or low sodium)
½ cup mirin
2 tbsp miso paste

1 piece of 2 x 2-inch fresh ginger root, peeled and cut into ⅛-inch slices
Handful of cilantro leaves
2 tbsp olive oil

Preheat oven to 400°F.

Mix soy sauce, mirin, miso paste, ginger slices, and cilantro in a bowl.

Place salmon filets into a gallon-size zipper storage bag.

Pour marinade into the storage bag and close.

Put in refrigerator, marinade for up to 2 hours.

Use an oven-proof skillet over medium-high heat. Heat 2 tbsp of olive oil, then carefully place each filet into skillet (skin side down if there is skin). Cook for about 5 minutes covered, then uncover and place the skillet into the oven for 10 minutes. Be careful removing it from the oven. Serve immediately. Garnish with fresh cilantro.

Notes: • *For easy clean up, line the baking sheet with aluminum foil and cook the salmon on the foil with edges rolled up slightly.* • *After cooking, it is easy to discard the foil and the pan should still be clean.*

Poached Salmon with Rosemary

Makes 4 servings | 515 calories per serving
Gluten-Free, Dairy-Free

4 salmon filets, 4–6 oz. apiece
4 sprigs fresh rosemary
4 half-slices fresh lemon
1 tsp olive oil

Place each filet skin-side down on a sheet of aluminum foil large enough to wrap the entire filet.

Place lemon and rosemary on the filet and drizzle ¼ tsp of the olive oil. Season with salt as needed.

Wrap each filet in foil and place in a baking pan in the oven at 350°F for 10–15 minutes.

To serve: remove from oven, unwrap the foil, and remove the lemon (do not squeeze it on the filet) and rosemary.

Serve with rice and your favorite steamed greens.

Notes: • Prep time is about 5 minutes for the salmon. • The tightly wrapped foil allows the filets to steam. • The rosemary (or other herbs of your choice) and the slice of lemon impart great flavor. • Since you are not squeezing the lemon on the fish, you avoid the acidity while enjoying the flavor—especially from the lemon rind that steams along with the filets. • If you like, drizzle olive oil on the fish before serving.

Risotto with Asparagus and Morels

Makes 2 servings | 300 calories per serving
Gluten-Free

1 cup Arborio rice

1 bunch asparagus (about 1 lb.) (peel the skin 3 inches below the head, cut to 1-inch lengths)

3 tbsp dried morel or porcini mushrooms (soak for 1 hour in water or vegetable stock)

2 cups vegetable stock (or 1 vegetable bouillon cube dissolved in 2 cups water)

2 bay leaves

4 sprigs thyme

2 tbsp Parmesan cheese (optional)

Salt to taste

Remove the reconstituted mushrooms from the water. Reserve the liquid.

Bring the vegetable stock (or vegetable bouillon cube and water), thyme, bay leaf, and reserved mushroom liquid to a boil. Cook for 5 minutes and remove bay leaf and thyme.

Cook the asparagus in the stock for a few minutes until al dente. Remove and cool immediately to preserve the green color. Reserve the stock.

Place the saucepan over medium heat. Add the rice and ½ cup of the stock. Bring to a simmer while continuing to stir.

Once the rice has absorbed nearly all the liquid, add another ½ cup of the stock, and continue to serve until the rice is creamy and al dente, about 20 minutes. Add more stock if the rice is too al dente or dry.

Add the asparagus, reconstituted mushrooms, and Parmesan cheese, and salt to taste. Serve immediately in a soup bowl.

Notes: • Dried morels are worth the trouble; morels are delicious and make this dish; this risotto is delicious and worth the trouble! • The morels are found in the grocery store dried; just reconstitute with water and then dry them. • Adding 2 tsp of Roquefort cheese to the risotto adds a twist to this classical dish. • The skin of the asparagus (about 3 to 4 inches below the head) tends to be fibrous. By peeling it you'll get a nice al dente crunch. If dicing, cut them on a bias.

Pan-Seared Soy-Glazed
Boneless-Skinless Chicken Thighs
Makes 4 servings | 350 calories per serving
Dairy Free

4 boneless, skinless chicken   thighs
1 tsp minced garlic (optional)
3 tbsp soy sauce
1 tsp brown sugar
Black pepper

3 tbsp rice wine/Chinese cooking
   wine (optional)
¼ tsp sesame oil
Splash of orange juice (optional)

Mix chicken thighs with marinade; let sit in bowl or zipper storage bag for one hour.

Heat skillet with 2 tbsp olive oil on medium-high, place the thighs in the skillet, (be careful of sizzle and oil splatter), cover, turn over after 5 minutes, then continue on medium heat for total of about 15–20 minutes, until golden brown.

Notes: • Your children will like this recipe as it is sweet and full of flavor. • Taking the skin off makes this dish healthier. • Serve with roasted veggies and a salad.

Chicken Cutlet with Prosciutto

Makes 2 servings | 270 calories per serving
Gluten-Free, Dairy Free

CHICKEN
1 chicken breast, boneless, skinless (12 oz.)
2 slices imported prosciutto, fat removed
2 tbsp olive oil
1 garlic clove (peeled and cut in half so it can be removed from pan after the oil is flavored) (optional)

VEGETABLES

1 cup zucchini (cut in half length-wise and sliced thin to create half-moon shapes)
2 cups green beans (ends trimmed)
2 cups chicken stock (or more if needed)
10 leaves fresh basil (washed, dried, leaves removed from the stems, chopped fine)

1 cup parsnip (peeled, cut in half lengthwise, and sliced thin)
½ cup carrots (peeled; diced into ⅓-inch cube)
¾ cup barley
Salt to taste

FOR THE CHICKEN

Split the whole breast in half and place the two sides flat on a cutting board. Slice horizontally to yield two thin cutlets.

Place one thin slice of prosciutto over one of the cutlets, and cover with the second chicken cutlet so that the prosciutto forms a thin layer in the middle.

Repeat with the second half-breast.

With a meat pounder or the side of a chef's knife, gently pound the cutlet so it adheres to the prosciutto.

Cover and refrigerate until needed.

FOR THE VEGETABLES

In a medium pot, bring the chicken stock to a boil. Add the green beans and cook until al dente, about 7 minutes. Drain and reserve the stock.

Cook the zucchini (about 30 seconds), parsnips (3–4 minutes), and carrots (4–5 minutes) the same way as the beans. Drain and reserve the stock each time.

Cook the barley in the same stock (about 15–20 minutes). When the barley is al dente, drain and store until needed.

DIRECTIONS

In a nonstick pan over medium heat, add the 2 tbsp olive oil and garlic. Cook until the garlic is golden brown. Remove the garlic and immediately place the chicken breast in the same oil. Cook for about 2–3 minutes, then flip. Cook for another minute or two. When done, remove and reserve. Do not discard the oil.

In the same pan, add the zucchini, parsnips, carrots, green beans, and barley. Heat on medium.

If the vegetables seem dry, add chicken stock. The barley tends to absorb a lot of liquid.

When the vegetables are warm, add salt as needed. Place the vegetables in a small mound on a plate. Cut the chicken cutlet in half lengthwise and place on top.

Garnish with chopped basil leaves.

Notes: • *The chicken stock evaporates as you cook the vegetables, so it's important to keep a little extra on hand. If the stock is flavorful enough, you can add water instead. • The chicken cutlet can be prepared up to one day in advance. Cover and refrigerate. • It is important to use a sharp chef's knife when slicing the basil, or it gets crushed and quickly turns black. • Barley takes 15–20 minutes to cook. You can substitute wheat berries, which take 30–40 minutes and have a slightly chewy consistency. • The garlic used in the oil should be discarded. It imparts a toasted garlic flavor without actually leaving garlic in the food. • Make sure you cook the vegetables one at a time, as their cooking times vary. • After cooking the vegetables, keep the stock to add flavor to a soup of your choice.*

Rice Porridge with Chicken

Makes 4 servings | 325 calories per serving
Gluten-Free, Dairy-Free

4 dried shiitake mushrooms
2 tbsp olive oil
1 tsp ginger minced
½ lb. ground chicken
4 cups chicken stock

2 cups cooked white rice
Salt to taste
2 tbsp chopped cilantro
1 tsp sesame oil (optional)

In warm water, soak mushrooms until soft.

Rinse the mushrooms and pat dry.

Remove the stems and thinly slice the caps.

Heat oil over medium-high heat. Add ginger and sauté for 1 minute. Add mushrooms and chicken, and sauté until chicken is browned. Set aside.

Heat chicken stock over medium-high heat until boiling.

Add rice, and bring to boil. Then reduce heat to low and cook until soft, about 15 minutes.

Add chicken and mushroom mixture, and cook another 5 minutes. Add salt to taste.

Pour into bowls, top with cilantro, drizzle with sesame oil, and serve.

Notes: • This is a common Taiwanese breakfast dish. • The chicken may be substituted with leftover vegetables, another meat, any fish or even leftover rice. • Every grandma in China and Japan will have her own version of this dish, and probably never measures anything. • Once you start, this may become one of your go-to recipes. • Have fun experimenting!

Salmon Fried Rice

Makes 4 servings | 375 calories per serving
Gluten-Free, Dairy-Free

4 tbsp olive oil
8 oz. smoked salmon
¼ cup fresh peas
¼ cup ¼-inch diced carrots

3 egg whites
1 egg yolk
3 cups of cooked rice
Salt to taste

Heat oil on medium-high, then add smoked salmon, and sauté until cooked through, breaking it into bite-sized pieces with spatula while stir-frying.

Add peas and carrots.

Whisk egg whites and egg yolk, then add to the pan.

Add rice and mix well.

Season with salt.

Notes: • Have leftover rice and don't know what to do with it? • This is a simple and quick dish that's made healthier with the addition of the omega-3 rich salmon.

Turkey and Mushrooms with Rice

Makes 6 servings | 450 calories per serving
Gluten-Free, Dairy-Free

6 dried shiitake mushrooms
3 tbsp olive oil
1 lb. ground turkey
1 tsp sugar
1 tbsp minced ginger
½ tsp Chinese spice blend
1 star anise

½ cup rice wine
2 cups water
½ cup tamari (soy sauce)
Cilantro (garnish)
Bean sprouts (garnish)
Julienned carrots (garnish)
Cooked Rice

In warm water, soak mushrooms until soft. Rinse the mushrooms and pat dry. Remove the stems and thinly slice the caps.

Heat oil over medium-high heat. Add ginger and sauté for 1 minute. Add mushrooms and turkey, and sauté until turkey is browned.

Add wine, soy sauce, water, sugar, and Chinese spice blend. Bring to boil, then lower to simmer for 45 minutes. Serve over rice, and garnish with cilantro, julienned carrots, and bean sprouts.

Notes: • You may use low-fat ground turkey meat instead of traditional ground pork.
• The vegetable garnish adds a crunchy freshness to the dish.

Tuscan-Style Pork Tenderloin

Makes 6 servings | 285 calories per serving
Gluten-Free

2 small-to-medium-sized pork tenderloins
1 tsp sea salt
2 to 3 tbsp olive oil
1 large bunch of fresh rosemary (roughly two handfuls)
1 to 1½ qts. of low-fat milk

Cut each of the pork tenderloins into three pieces, and salt all sides.

Heat oil in soup pot on medium-high, and brown the six pork pieces.

When pork pieces are browned, lower heat to medium, and add the rosemary.

Cover the rosemary and the meat with milk; it will take about a quart, possibly more.

Bring to a slow, bubbling boil for 45 minutes.

Remove the meat and slice, serving each portion with some of the intact rosemary stems.

Notes: • This dish makes the entire house smell wonderful because of the rosemary. • Use fresh rosemary; dried will not do. • Serve with roasted mashed root veggies, sautéed string beans or roasted asparagus with black olives.

Basil Chicken

Makes 6 servings | 325 calories per serving
Gluten-Free, Dairy-Free

¼ cup sesame oil (use extra virgin olive oil if sesame oil is a trigger food)

10 slices ginger

1 cup rice wine (preferably Shaoxing or dry sherry)

1 cup tamari (soy sauce)

2 whole star anise (or 1 tbsp anise seed)

1 tbsp honey

2 lbs. chicken breast, chopped into bite-size chunks

1 bunch basil

Steamed white rice, for serving

Heat oil over medium-high heat, add ginger, and cook until fragrant, about 1 minute.

Add chicken pieces and brown for 1 to 2 minutes.

Add rice wine, soy sauce, star anise, and honey, and bring to a boil. Reduce heat to a simmer for 15 minutes or until chicken is cooked through.

Stir in basil, and remove from heat. Serve over rice.

Notes: • This is a traditional Taiwanese dish that is often called "three cup chicken," with tremendous variations from family to family. • The "three cup" refers to the fact that this dish is usually made with equal parts rice wine, soy sauce, and sesame oil. • Note: Sesame oil can be a reflux trigger for some people.

Steamed Halibut with Prosciutto

Makes 4 servings | 385 calories per serving
Gluten-Free, Dairy-Free

1 lb. halibut
½ tsp salt
½ tsp rice wine (optional)
5 dried shiitake mushrooms
4 tbsp olive oil

4 slices of ginger
10 slices of prosciutto
10 slices of canned bamboo shoots
1 cup chicken or vegetable stock
2 tbsp cilantro, chopped

Marinade halibut in salt and rice wine for 10 minutes.

Soak mushrooms in warm water until soft. Rinse the mushrooms, and pat dry. Remove the stems, and thinly slice the caps.

Heat oil over medium-high heat, add ginger, and sauté for 1 minute. Add mushrooms, prosciutto, and bamboo shoots, and sauté for 1 minute.

Add halibut and chicken stock, and cook until chicken stock is reduced and fish is cooked through.

Top with cilantro and serve.

Notes: • *The saltiness of the prosciutto and earthiness of the shiitake mushrooms adds complexity to this flavorful dish.* • *Serve alone or with a bowl of steamed rice.*

Turkey Burger Salad with Black Olives and Avocado

Makes 4 servings | 275 calories per serving
Gluten-Free, Dairy-Free

1 lb. of ground turkey meat (preferably 93–97% fat, as 99% fat-free can be too dry) made into four patties

½ tsp sea salt

2 heads of romaine lettuce, clean and cut or torn into 2–3-inch pieces

1 medium-sized can of small-pitted black olives

1 tsp of balsamic vinegar

2 tbsp of extra virgin olive oil

1 avocado peeled and sliced

Salt and cook turkey burgers on grill or on the stove top in a covered fry pan on medium to medium-high heat 4–5 minutes per side.

After cooking, put burgers aside until cool enough to break into bite-sized pieces.

Place lettuce, olives, oil, and vinegar in a large salad bowl and toss.

Finally, add burger and avocado on top.

Notes: • Turkey burgers are a good source of protein. • The black olives and the avocado give a nice contrasting texture and flavor. This salad can be enhanced any number of ways. You can add sautéed mushrooms if you want to leave off the avocado.

Pasta with Zucchini, Shrimp, and Basil

Makes 6 servings | 460 calories per serving
Gluten-Free

1 lb. spaghetti (or if you are gluten-free, get gluten-free white-rice spaghetti pasta)

3 to 4 medium-sized zucchinis, sliced the long way and then into ¼-inch half-moon slices

½ tsp of sea salt

4 tbsp of olive oil

1½ to 2 lbs. of shrimp (fresh or frozen/cooked) peeled and deveined

¾ cup of fresh basil leaves, stems removed

Freshly grated Parmesan cheese for garnish (optional); if you are dairy-free, then no cheese

Get all of the ingredients ready at the start, because the sauce will take about the same time as the pasta to cook. If the shrimp are frozen, defrost them in cold water, and then dry them.

Fill large pasta pot ⅔ with water, and put on high heat.

When the water comes to a vigorous, rolling boil, put the pasta in.

Start the sauce when the pasta goes into the boiling water.

Salt the zucchini.

In large saucepan, pour half of olive oil, and on high heat, brown the zucchini slices, turning them with a spatula. Try not to "boil" them; that is, a big pan and high heat is best.

When the zucchini is almost done, add the shrimp and basil. Add more olive oil, if needed.

When the pasta is done, drain and serve in individual bowls.

Top with the shrimp and zucchini sauce and Parmesan.

Notes: • *This is an example of a reflux-friendly, gluten-free spaghetti dish that is easy and fast. The rice pasta is remarkably delicious; it also reheats well.* • *Don't worry about how much olive oil you use; it typically does not cause reflux. (And, by the way, if you use butter, olive oil always makes for a great substitute. You can use it on every-thing—pasta, meat, potatoes, fish, veggies, rice, etc.)* • *Consider variations of this dish: Include other vegetables: carrots, spinach; really anything will do. And if you have left-over meat or fish, you can use that instead of shrimp. It can even be prepared with cod, snow peas, and cilantro.*

Poached Arctic Char with Dill

Makes 4 servings | 210 calories per serving
Gluten-Free, Dairy-Free

1 lb. Arctic char
1 cup chicken or vegetable stock
1 to 2 tsp olive oil
1 tsp sea salt
2 tsp of fresh dill, stems removed and finely cut

Cut the fish in half, so that it will fit neatly in your pan, or you may cut it into individual servings.

Cover both sides of fish lightly with olive oil and then the salt.

Heat the pan on medium-high heat, and then add the fish, skin side up.

Sauté for 2–3 minutes until there is some sizzle.

Add the chicken broth and half of the dill.

When the stock is boiling lightly and steaming, cover the pan with the lid or foil. (Observe for a minute. You can see if the heat is too high when the steam around the edges of the pan becomes excessive).

Cook for 12–18 minutes, until the fish skin peels off with ease. That's how you will know it's done.

Plate, and garnish with the rest of the fresh dill.

Notes: • *To cook this fish properly, you will need a shallow stovetop pan with a cover.* • *If you don't have a cover for your most suitable fry pan, you can cover with tinfoil for the poaching of the fish.* • *Arctic char is a delicious, light, flavorful, and delicate fish with exceptionally pleasing texture.* • *You may substitute any other fish-friendly spice if you prefer (like basil).* • *This Arctic char dish goes extremely well with the rice with cumin and turmeric dish on page 127, as well as with sautéed or roasted vegetables such as eggplant, string beans, or asparagus.* • *This same dish can be made with salmon that is not too thick (less than 1½ inches).*

Chicken Schnitzel

Makes 4 servings | 321 calories per serving

1 package of skinless boneless chicken breasts
2 tbsp olive oil
1 cup plain or seasoned bread crumbs
1 egg

Pound the chicken breasts until they are very thin.

Beat an egg in a small bowl and dip the pounded chicken in the egg to create a small film over it.

Place bread crumbs in a plate. You can use seasoned bread crumbs for more flavor.

Dip the coated chicken in the bread crumbs and coat both sides of the chicken.

Heat a pan with 1 tbsp of olive oil until sizzling.

Place the chicken in the pan and fry until it starts getting dark, then flip sides until well done.

Set aside to cool on a plate with a paper towel to soak up the oil

Serve warm with couscous and steamed asparagus.

Notes: • *Most kids enjoy doing the pounding of the chicken breasts for the schnitzel.*
• *If you don't have a meat pounder, you can place clear plastic wrap around a wine (or other full) bottle and use the side of it. (No, you will not break the bottle unless you are pounding wildly.)*

Steamed Sea Bass with Ginger and Soy

Makes 4 servings | 380 calories per serving
Gluten-Free, Dairy-Free

2 lbs. sea bass filet (or any flaky
  white fish)
2 tsp sea salt
1-inch ginger, peeled and cut into
  matchsticks
1½ tbsp rice wine (or any cooking
  wine)

2 tbsp soy sauce
4 tsp toasted sesame oil (optional)
1 tbsp olive oil
½ cup fresh cilantro sprigs

Salt both sides of filet.

Scatter ginger over top of fish.

Drizzle rice wine over the fish, and place on a heat-proof dish for steaming. Place in steamer and cover. Steam for 10–15 minutes. Pour water out of the dish.

Drizzle soy sauce over the fish.

Heat toasted sesame oil and olive oil over medium-high heat until they begin to smoke.

Carefully pour oil on top of the fish.

Garnish with cilantro and serve immediately.

Notes: • A firm, white-fleshed fish, such as cod or halibut, may be substituted for the sea bass. • Sesame oil may be a reflux trigger for some people.

Stir-Fry Rice Noodles with Vegetables

Makes 4 servings | 300 calories per serving
Vegetarian, Gluten-Free, Dairy-Free

½ lb. dried rice noodles
2 tbsp olive oil
2 tbsp ginger, minced
4 shiitake mushrooms, sliced thin
1 carrot, cut into matchsticks
1 cup choy sum (or bok choy), cut
  into 1-inch slivers

½ cup basil, chopped
2 tbsp tamari (soy sauce)
2 tsp palm sugar
1 tbsp Shaoxing wine (or sherry)
⅓ cup seaweed or vegetable stock

Pour boiling water over rice noodles in a bowl. Let soak 2–5 minutes or until noodles are soft.

Do NOT over soak. Drain, rinse in cold water, and set aside.

In hot wok or skillet, add oil and ginger. Stir-fry 1 minute over medium-high heat.

Add shiitake, carrots, choy sum, and basil. Continue stir-frying for 3 minutes.

Add the rest of ingredients and bring to boil, stirring constantly.

Add the drained rice noodles, and mix gently. Serve very hot.

Notes: • *Rice noodles have a wonderful texture, are gluten-free, and have been made in China and Southeast Asia for millennia.* • *This dish is known as Chow Fun in China and Pad Kee Mao in Thailand.*

Clams with Basil and Ginger

Makes 4 servings | 170 calories per serving
Gluten-Free, Dairy-Free

1 tbsp olive oil
2 cloves garlic
1-inch ginger, peeled and cut into
   matchsticks
1 lb. clams
1 tbsp rice wine

2 tbsp tamari (soy sauce)
1 tsp sugar
2 tbsp water
Pinch of salt to taste
½ cup basil leaves

Heat oil on medium-high heat, add garlic and ginger, and stir fry until fragrant for 1 minute. Fish out and discard the garlic clove.

Add clams. Stir-fry on high heat until shells start to open.

Add rice wine, soy sauce, sugar, and water. Stir-fry until the sauce is almost dry, and season to taste with salt.

Add basil and serve.

Notes: • This healthy and flavorful dish is very quick to make. • The fragrant basil makes a huge difference. • Omit garlic if you think that it might be a reflux trigger for you or someone else in your family.

SNACKS AND
HORS D'OEUVRES

Garbanzo Bean Spread

Makes 24 servings | 50 calories per serving

1¼ cups garbanzo beans (soaked in
    water for a couple of hours or
    overnight in the refrigerator)
3 qts. chicken stock
2 oz. (4 slices) prosciutto

1 bay leaf
2 branches fresh thyme
2 tbsp sesame seeds, toasted golden
    brown
Salt to taste

Drain the water from the beans and place them with 2½ quarts of the chicken stock in a medium pot.

Add the slices of prosciutto, the bay leaf, and the thyme. Place a cover over ¾ of the pot and simmer about 2 hours.

If the stock reduces to a level below the beans, add more stock to cover.

When the beans are soft, drain them. Remove the bay leaves, thyme, and prosciutto. Cool and place in a food processor with the sesame seeds, and process until smooth.

Add salt and chicken stock as needed for the desired consistency.

Serve cold with toast points, oven-toasted corn chips, or small wedges of flatbread.

Notes: • You can simplify the procedure by using an 8 oz. can of chickpeas. If you do so, rinse twice under cold water and process in a food processor until smooth. It will save 2 hours, but you sacrifice some flavor. If you add salt while cooking the beans, the cooking time will be lengthened by several hours, as the outside skin of the chickpeas will not soften. • For added flavor, the prosciutto can be processed with the beans (it will not be as smooth, though). • The traditional hummus recipe calls for tahini, which is a paste of roasted sesame seeds. Since it is not always available, we've substituted freshly roasted sesame seeds.

No-Alarm Mexican Salsa

Makes 20 servings | 30 calories per serving
Vegetarian, Gluten-Free, Dairy-Free

½ cup corn kernels (fresh or canned)
½ cup cucumber (washed, cut in half, seeds removed, and diced into ¼-inch cubes)
½ cup banana (peeled and diced into ¼-inch cubes)
½ cup pineapple (fresh, peeled, cut in half lengthwise, then in quarters, core removed, and diced into ¼-inch cubes)
½ cup canned black beans (rinsed and drained)
1 avocado, sliced and diced
Optional: ½ cup honeydew (skin and seeds removed, then diced into ¼-inch cubes)

¼ tsp fresh ginger, grated
½ tsp ground cumin (best if whole cumin is roasted in a pan and ground when needed)
2 tbsp fresh parsley (washed, stems removed, dried, and chopped fine)
2 tbsp fresh cilantro (washed, stems removed, dried, and chopped coarse)
2 tbsp olive oil
¼ cup pineapple juice
1 tsp salt, or more to taste

Place the corn, cucumber, banana, pineapple, black beans, honeydew, ginger, cumin, parsley, cilantro, olive oil, and pineapple in a bowl.

Mix thoroughly and season with salt.

Add the avocado last, as it can easily become mashed.

Serve immediately before the bright green color of the herbs fades.

Notes: • *If you don't mind the herbs turning a darker green, you can let it sit for half an hour, allowing the flavors to blend* • *Fresh corn tastes especially good during the summer season, when it is sweet* • *This recipe is best served cold. If you don't serve immediately, keep refrigerated, or the chlorophyll will blacken.* • *This salsa is delicious with fish.*

Sweet Potato Bites

Makes 8 servings | 65 calories per serving
Vegetarian, Dairy-Free

2 large sweet potatoes, (peeled, rinsed, and diced into 1-inch cubes)
1 tbsp low-sodium soy sauce
1 tbsp honey
5 sprigs thyme (washed, stems removed, and chopped fine)
Nonstick spray (about ½ tsp)

In a bowl, mix the soy sauce, thyme, and honey.

Add the cubed potatoes and let stand for 1 minute.

Drain the potatoes, dry slightly with a paper towel, and place in the pan in a single layer.

Brown all sides and, if not tender, finish in a 350°F oven for about 10 minutes.

You can serve the potatoes in a flat ceramic dish with toothpicks.

Notes: • If the potatoes are getting too brown in the pan, lower the heat and finish in the oven at 350°F. • To speed up the cooking process, cover with a lid so the heat is dispersed more evenly throughout the pan. • If you'd like this snack a little sweeter, you can pour extra honey or maple syrup over the potatoes.

Skillet Cornbread

Makes 4 servings | 175 calories per serving
Gluten-Free, Dairy-Free

DRY MIX
1 cup yellow cornmeal
1 cup flour
1 tbsp baking powder
½ tsp sea salt

WET MIX
1¼ cups soy milk
3 tbsp olive oil
2 tsp maple syrup

Preheat a 9-inch cast iron skillet in a 425°F oven for ½ hour.

Whisk together the dry mix in a bowl, and put aside.

Put all the wet mix ingredients in a blender, and blend until smooth.

Add wet to dry. Mix lightly, but do not over mix!

Pour batter into a well-oiled, HOT cast iron skillet (a cast iron skillet will provide an ideal texture). Cook on stove a few minutes over medium-low heat until bubbles begin to appear on the surface. Then bake for 30 minutes or until the toothpick comes out clean.

Notes: • Option 1: Add 1 red apple, cored, peeled, and grated, to the wet mix. • Option 2: Sauté 1 ear of corn, shucked, and 1 red pepper, chopped in 1 tbsp olive oil for 3 minutes. Add this to the batter and then cook as directed above.

Marbled Tea Eggs

Makes 6 servings | 70 calories per serving
Gluten-Free, Dairy-Free

6 eggs, hard boiled
¾ cup tamari (soy sauce)
1 cup water

½-inch ginger, sliced
2 black tea bags (optional)
½ teaspoon Chinese spice powder

Crack the hard-boiled eggs well, but do not peel. This will give the eggs a mottled look.

Add the eggs to the pot with tamarind, water, sliced ginger, black tea bags, and Chinese spice powder. Make sure liquid completely covers the eggs. Add more water if needed to cover the eggs.

Simmer over low heat for 25 minutes. Let it steep for 30 minutes, then cool.

Crack open, peel the eggs, and slice into wedges to serve.

Notes: • This is a famous Chinese street food. • The staining and cracking process creates a beautiful marbled effect. • Serve them as a snack or a whimsical addition for breakfast or brunch.

Royal Caviar Egg Treat

Makes 1 serving | 170 calories per serving
Gluten-Free, Dairy-Free

3 jumbo hard boiled eggs
1 jar of salmon roe (caviar)

Peel the eggs and break them in half, dumping out the yolks.

Line up the six half-eggs, leaning on each other so that they stand up. (Using a sharp knife you can cut the tip off the pointy end, so that they stand on their own.)

Using a knife finely chop one yolk, and with the knife place some yolk in each egg-half.

Top each liberally with caviar.

Notes: • You don't have to use jumbo eggs, but the yolk is generally the same size in dif-ferent-sized eggs so the jumbos will have proportionally more egg white. • For easy-to-peel hard boiled eggs, don't use recently bought eggs; eggs that are at least a week old simply peel better. • After boiling, cool them quickly in the refrigerator. • Relatively inexpensive salmon roe is great; don't buy expensive caviar for this yummy snack. • If you are serving caviar eggs to company, cut the pointy bottoms square so they stand up straight on a plate, and use a cocktail napkin or a small doily to keep the eggs from sliding around.

Turkey Lettuce Cup with Pine Nuts

Makes 8 servings | 200 calories per serving
Dairy-Free

2 tsp olive oil
1-inch piece of ginger, diced
1 lb. ground turkey
2 tbsp oyster sauce
2 tbsp tamari (soy sauce)

¼ cup green beans, finely sliced
¾ cup pine nuts
Salt to taste
8 iceberg lettuce leaves
¼ cup shredded carrots

Heat oil in large sauté pan on medium-high heat, add ginger and cook until fra-grant.

Add ground turkey and sauté until turkey is browned.

Add oyster sauce, soy sauce, green beans, pine nuts, and salt to taste. Mix well for 2 minutes.

Serve in lettuce cups topped with shredded carrots.

Notes: • These wraps are delicious and bursting with flavor. • The clean crispness of the lettuce and the crunch of pine nuts play well with the saltiness of the turkey mixture. • Can be made into beautifully tantalizing bite-size appetizers (by trimming lettuce to desired size and filling with turkey mixture) or served family style, letting everyone make their own.

Parmesan and Dill Popcorn

Serves 5 | 65 calories per serving
Gluten-Free

1 cup popping-corn kernels
1 tbsp olive oil
1 tbsp grated Parmesan cheese
2 tbsp fresh dill (washed, stems removed, and chopped fine)

Heat a pan that is large enough to hold the corn in a single layer over medium heat.

Add the oil and the corn and stir until the corn starts to pop (about 3–5 minutes).

Cover the pan and lower the temperature.

Once the popcorn has stopped popping, remove from heat immediately.

Pour the corn into a bowl, then sprinkle with the grated Parmesan and fine-chopped dill.

Stir the cheese and herbs to mix evenly.

Serve promptly.

Notes: • Make sure the pan is preheated (hot) before adding the oil and corn. Remove the corn that has not popped. • You can omit the dill or replace it with another herb of your choice.

DESSERTS

Kick-A** Carrot Cookies

Makes 3 dozen cookies | 65 calories per cookie
Vegetarian, Dairy-Free

1 cup oats
1 cup flour
1 tsp cinnamon
1 tsp baking powder
½ tsp baking soda

¼ tsp salt
½ cup maple syrup
½ cup grape seed oil
1 cup grated carrots
½ cup dried cherries (see Notes)

Preheat oven to 375°F.

In one bowl, combine oats, flour, cinnamon, baking powder, baking soda, and salt.

In a separate bowl, whisk together maple syrup and oil.

Add carrots and dried fruit to this mix, and blend well.

Pour the wet mix over the dry mix and gently combine. Do not over mix, or the cookies will be rubbery.

These cookies only bake well if they are small.

Drop 1 tsp of the mixture on an oiled baking sheet, with each cookie 2 inches apart.

Bake at 375°F for 10 minutes.

Be careful not to overcook, as they burn easily.

Notes: • For the picky eaters in your home, why not sneak a little carrot into their diet with this amazing cookie recipe? • For a fun variation, dried cherries can be replaced by currants, raisins, dried blueberries, dried cranberries, or a combination.

Natural Fruit Mold

Makes 4 servings | 70 calories per serving
Vegetarian, Gluten-Free, Dairy-Free

2 cups water
1 cup blueberry juice
2 tsp kanten (agar) powder
Fresh seasonal fruit, sliced
Seasonal berries

In a saucepan, heat up water and juice, add kanten powder with a whisk, and constantly stir to dissolve.

Bring the mixture to a boil, lower heat, and cook, stirring constantly for 3 minutes.

Pour the kanten mixture in a pan.

Decorate with fresh fruit slices and berries.

Let set 2 hours; chill before serving.

Notes: • Originally from Japan, this is a very refreshing summer dish and is quite simple and inexpensive to prepare. • Kanten has an immediate cooling effect on the body and is also very good for digestion. • Multiple layers of kanten can be prepared for a very beautiful plate. After you prepare one layer, let it fully set, and then prepare the second layer. Use different juices with different colors to create a rainbow effect.

Banana Pistachio Ice Cream

Makes approx. 1 quart | 150 calories per large scoop
Vegetarian, Gluten-Free, Dairy-Free

½ cup raw unsalted pistachios
2 cups water
½ cup maple syrup
4 ripe bananas
½ tsp cinnamon

Place all ingredients in a blender, and puree until totally smooth.

Add this puree to an ice cream maker, and churn until frozen.

Note: • This ice cream can be can be made with milk instead of water.

Ginger-Carrot Ice Pop

Makes 6 servings | 150 calories per serving
Vegetarian, Gluten-Free, Dairy-Free

2 tbsp honey
2 cups carrot juice
2 tsp ginger juice

Mix all ingredients and pour into ice pop mold. Insert sticks and freeze until set.

Notes: • *It doesn't get any better than this, a healthy and cheap alternative to store-bought ice pops for kids.* • *These ice-pop molds are great for all types of frozen fruit and fruit juice desserts.*

Quick Banana Sorbet

Makes 6 servings | 45 calories per serving
Vegetarian, Gluten-Free, Dairy-Free

3 bananas, peeled
1 tbsp ginger (peeled and grated fine)
⅛ tsp ground cardamom

2 tbsp honey
¼ tsp salt
3 cups ice

Place the bananas, ginger, cardamom, honey, and salt in the blender.

Blend on high until smooth.

Add ice and blend until creamy. Add more ice as needed.

Serve immediately or store in freezer.

Notes: • *To make this sorbet, it's best to use a heavy-duty blender with a tamper that allows you to push the ice cubes down toward the blender blades.* • *If an air pocket forms around the blades, stop the blender, stir, and start again.*

Pear Cardamom Sorbet

Makes 15 servings | 150 calories per serving
Gluten-Free

2 lbs. fresh Bartlett pears (washed, peeled, halved, cored, and cut into 1-inch pieces)
3 cups water
1½ cups honey
½ tsp salt

1 tsp vanilla extract
1 tsp grated ginger (peeled and grated fine)
⅛ tsp ground cardamom
2 cups milk

In a large saucepan, add to water pears, honey, salt, vanilla, ginger, and cardamom.

Bring to a boil, and simmer for 20 minutes or until pears are tender.

Using a hand blender, mix until smooth.

Cool and place in ice cube trays. Freeze overnight.

Notes: • Try to use very ripe pears. • Leave the skin on for the vitamins, but remember to wash the pears thoroughly. • If you are using canned pears, make the sorbet the same day; place the drained pears in a blender and add the honey, salt, vanilla, ginger, cardamom, and ice. Blend and add milk to the desired consistency.

Watermelon Sorbet

Serves 4 | 15 calories per serving
Vegetarian, Gluten-Free, Dairy-Free

4 cups watermelon puree
1 tbsp lemon zest

Puree watermelon in a high-speed blender, and add lemon juice.

Freeze in an ice cream maker according to manufacturer's instructions.

Note: • It would be hard to find something more refreshing and quenching in the summer than this insanely simple-to-create dish.

APPENDIX A

Medical and Surgical Options for Infants and Children with Reflux

Upon consulting this section, you have presumably exhausted all of the treatments recommended in this book, changing your child's diet, giving smaller feedings, or having her sleep on an upright incline. Should reflux persist despite your best efforts, that should be a red flag indicating something more may be needed. We reiterate: in these cases, not one, but two specialists may be needed: one to evaluate the respiratory tract (an otolaryngologist) and another to evaluate the digestive tract (a gastroenterologist).

For most children with recalcitrant reflux, the first medical line of defense is an acid-suppression medication from the H2-receptor blocker (H2A) group such as ranitidine (Zantac), famotidine (Pepcid), or cimetidine (Tagamet). These are the safest and best-tolerated anti-reflux medications available. They come in liquid form and may be administered with meals and at bedtime. There are other groups of acid-suppressive medications that should be considered "second-line," as they come with a variety of drawbacks and side effects. More on these to follow.

If your pediatrician has put your child on anti-reflux medicine, that decision is ultimately between you and your doctor. Most infants and children with reflux, however, don't actually need to be on medicine, or at the very least, they don't have to be on medicine for long.

This appendix covers a few things that you should know about the different classes of reflux medications, including some of their potential benefits and side effects. This information is particularly important today, because all of the different types of medicines used for reflux are sold over-the-counter; that is, you can get them without a doctor's prescription.

It is beyond the scope of this book to recommend anti-reflux medication; however, we will briefly discuss how they are different and suggest which we believe are the safest in our medical practices.

Commonly Used Anti-Reflux Medications

Class of Medication	Examples (not inclusive)
Alginates	Gaviscon
Antacids	Tums and Rolaids
	Milk of Magnesia
	Maalox
	Mylanta
	Digel
H2-Antogonists (H2As)	Zantac (ranitidine)
	Pepcid (famotidine)
	Tagamet (cimetidine)
Proton Pump Inhibitors (PPIs)	Prilosec (omeprazole)
	Protonix (pantaprozole)
	Prevacid (lansoprazole)
	Aciphex (rabeprazole)
	Dexilant (dexlansoprazole)
	Zegerid (omeprazole/ bicarbonate)
	Nexium (esomeprazole)
Mucosal Protectants	Carafate (sucralfate)
Prokinetic Agent	Bethanechol (Urecholine)

Alginates. One of the most popular and safest anti-reflux medications in Europe, Gaviscon, is made out of seaweed extract. It forms a gooey "raft" in the top of the stomach that helps block reflux from occurring in the first place. In our opinion, American Gaviscon "Extra Strength" is not as effective as the European brand; we recommend the liquid "Gaviscon Advance Aniseed" that can be purchased online. (The "Extra Strength" is not the same product as the Gaviscon "Advance," the superior product.) Gaviscon may be taken after meals and before bed to help prevent reflux. Talk to your doctor before starting this or any other any medication.

Antacids. Over-the-counter antacids are mostly used by adults with heartburn and indigestion and are not commonly used by children. Of the antacids on the market, we have no preference, and they all appear to be relatively safe.

H2-Antogonists (H2As). This class of acid-suppressive, anti-reflux medication is the safest group of medications for which medical anti-reflux treatment is indicated. H2As come in a liquid as well as pill form. They are usually given 30 minutes before meals and bedtime. H2A side effects are uncommon but include dizziness, elevated heart rate, headaches, and rashes. H2As are safe enough that they are sometimes used during pregnancy.

Proton Pump Inhibitors (PPIs). This is the strongest class of acid-suppressive medication. You may have seen them advertised extensively on television, in print media, and online. Several brands are sold over-the-counter. Because of their side effects, the benefit of these medications is controversial in children (and in adults). Try to avoid injudicious use of PPIs for your kids. Do not buy them over-the-counter, and use PPIs only under a physician's supervision. Even then, ask how long the child will be taking them. In children, PPIs can cause diarrhea, abdominal pain, bloating, vomiting, headache, and rashes. If your child needs to be on a PPI based on your ENT, lung, or primary doctor's clinical assessment, make sure that the child is evaluated by a gastroenterologist to monitor long-term side effects and to ensure that there are no other medical issues that can lead to the reflux symptoms that are being treated.

Mucosal Protectants Sucralfate (carafate) is supposed to protect the esophageal lining from damage caused by reflux. It is not used in children very often, and it requires a doctor's prescription.

Prokinetic Medications. Prokinetic agents are used to increase the function of a "lazy" esophagus that doesn't empty well. These drugs have a lot of side effects and should be generally avoided unless your pediatrician or pediatric gastroenterologist recommends them.

In our practices, when medication is needed, we generally use H2As and sometimes we prescribe PPIs. Remember, healthy diet and lifestyle are far more effective treatments for most infants, children, and adults than medication.

Anti-Reflux Surgery

For serious refluxers, particularly those with potentially life-threatening reflux conditions, there is a surgical option: fundoplication.[55] The name of this procedure is almost self-explanatory. In fundoplication, the fundus (the dome of the stomach) is plicated (sewn) around the esophagus to create a new, tight lower esophageal sphincter (LES) valve.

Most fundoplication procedures are highly successful and eradicate reflux by creating a robust band of healthy tissue that allows food to get into the stomach, but not back up and out again. For children whose reflux is causing serious respiratory disease, fundoplication may inevitably be the best treatment option; however, with it comes risks that you and your surgeon must weigh before proceeding with such a definitive procedure.

It May Not Be Reflux: Serious Medical Conditions that May Mimic or Be Complicated by Reflux

By now, we hope you are inspired and believe in your ability to help your child become healthier simply by eating a nutritious, low-fat, low-acid diet. In earlier sections, we have explained why acid reflux in children is under-diagnosed and usually not "fixed" by simply giving children medications to decrease stomach acid. There are other conditions, however, for which a healthy diet alone may not be the fix, and which require medical or even surgical treatment. Because these problems may be more serious than everyday reflux, affected children must be diagnosed and managed by doctors.

This section is not encyclopedic; that is, not all possible diagnoses are included. We have, instead, selected those problems we have experienced first-hand in our practices, believing these to be the more common conditions that require medical intervention. The purpose of this chapter is to alert you to warning signs that signal serious diagnoses that can be potentially life threatening.

Potentially Serious Signs and Symptoms

- Fever
- Seizures
- Turning blue
- Choking episodes
- Stopping breathing
- Difficulty swallowing
- Worsening noisy breathing
- Change in alertness or lethargy
- Chest retractions on inspiration
- Compromised breathing (struggling to get air)
- Excessive spitting up or frequent vomiting

- Projectile vomiting or vomiting of bile
- Stomach swelling or tenderness
- Blood in the vomit or the stool
- Failure to thrive (meet expected weight gain)
- Documented or suspected genetic syndrome

> **If you're concerned about your child's breathing or feeding, see a physician without delay.**

In general, the first line of specialists for persistent or worrisome breathing problems are pediatric otolaryngologists (ENTs) and then pulmonologists (lung doctors), if needed. For unremitting or serious digestive problems such as projectile vomiting, a pediatric gastroenterologist may be consulted. These consultations will usually be requested by your pediatrician, but you can advocate for your child and ask for a specialist referral yourself.

Two groups of overlapping conditions are discussed in this book: respiratory and digestive problems. In some infants, failure to thrive—to gain weight and develop in a timely fashion—may be due to respiratory and/or digestive problems. There are, however, other causes of failure to thrive to consider.

Before proceeding to discuss these "other" diagnoses, it is important to point out that there is still an important relationship between reflux and respiratory diseases. Indeed, we believe that most respiratory diseases in children are either caused by reflux *or* are exacerbated and/or complicated by reflux in tandem with a coincident medical condition.

Sometimes, the effect of reflux is more than additive (two plus two equals four), it may act like a catalyst multiplying the effects of a disease severalfold. This means that reflux is acting like an accelerant. See an interesting case example on page 181 to understand how reflux control can be a crucial factor in achieving a successful outcome when it occurs with another serious concomitant disease.

As another example, in the authors' experience, reflux is a crucial factor in subglottic stenosis. Subglottic stenosis is scarring that causes narrowing of the breathing tube just below the vocal cords. Subglottic stenosis causes persistent noisy breathing.

Subglottic stenosis can be congenital; that is, some children are born with it. Most cases, however, are caused by having a breathing tube in place for medical purposes. Regardless of the origin, swelling from reflux can worsen the problem by causing persistent inflammation and subsequent scar formation in the affected tissues. Reflux should be ruled-out in all cases of subglottic stenosis, as it can worsen or even be the root cause of the disease. This topic is further discussed below.

We otolaryngologists (ENT specialists) work very closely with other pediatric subspecialty colleagues in managing complex patients. Some of our patients have multiple underlying medical conditions involving problems of the heart, lungs, nervous system, and bones. Today, many children's hospitals in the United States have multidisciplinary aerodigestive (breathing and digestive system) clinics to manage children who have complicated breathing and digestive problems.

For patients referred for recurrent croup and/or chronic cough who do not respond to reflux management, we may recommend an examination under anesthesia, where, in the operating room, an airway endoscopy can be performed. Such examinations are most often purely diagnostic. There is no one-size-fits-all approach to aerodigestive problems in pediatric patients, but vigilance and attention to detail, including consideration of alternative diagnoses, is required.

While beyond the scope of this book to discuss in detail, there are a host of relevant congenital and acquired conditions that have many serious negative impacts on children's well-being. Some affect the respiratory tract, digestive tract, or both. Many of these conditions cause or exacerbate reflux, while some are the direct result of reflux. Shown in the list below are the most common of these conditions, some of which can be life threatening. This list is not intended to be comprehensive.

Serious and Life-Threatening Medical Conditions That May Mimic or Be Complicated by Reflux

Airway and Lung Problems
Laryngomalacia
Laryngospasm
Brief resolved unexplained event (BRUE)
Sudden infant death syndrome (SIDS)
Foreign body in the airway

Allergy and asthma
Aspiration (multifactorial causes)
Glottic and subglottic stenosis
Broncho-pulmonary dysplasia
Cystic fibrosis

Gastrointestinal Problems
Constipation
Pyloric stenosis
Eosinophilic esophagitis
Malrotation of the bowel

Combined Gastrointestinal and Airway Problems
Recurrent pneumonia
Tracheoesophageal fistula and esophageal atresia
Congenital diaphragmatic hernia
Cricopharyngeal achalasia

Cardiac and Neurological Problems

Reflux Can Make Laryngomalacia Much Worse

Reflux is a problem in most babies with laryngomalacia because it causes swelling in the area of the voice box and can cause the baby to have less sensation in that area—causing more swallowing difficulties. Treating reflux significantly improves the condition.

Airway and Lung Problems

If your child is having difficult or labored breathing, or if her breathing rate appears elevated, consult your pediatrician or an ENT doctor immediately. While reflux can cause some babies to have difficulty breathing, and vice versa, breathing hard can cause reflux to worsen. This does not mean that you should just spend the next three months monitoring your child's diet and hoping for the best.

Doctors must first establish that there is no underlying problem with the voice box (larynx), windpipe (trachea), lungs, or stomach. Sometimes, if the stomach is getting very full, it can put pressure on the lungs and cause a baby to have breathing difficulties. Reflux can occur, but other underlying causes need to be explored by your doctor. Your pediatrician should know how to further evaluate this situation.

Laryngomalacia (Mostly Affects Infants)

If your baby is having noisy breathing on inhalation and sounds like a squeaky toy or produces loud hiccups, your pediatrician should be informed. It is up to you and your pediatrician to determine if an evaluation by an ENT specialist is needed. Noisy breathing on the inhalation (inspiratory noises, inspiratory stridor) is most commonly a result of being born with floppiness in the cartilages that sit on the top of the voice box. This relatively common and benign condition is called laryngomalacia, and it is often associated with reflux. If a baby is working hard to breathe, s/he may reflux more, which can result in swelling of the structures above the esophagus, including the vocal cords. When the breathing structures get more swollen, it gets more difficult to breath and they become even noisier. This becomes a vicious cycle.

Normally, the epiglottis functions by closing over the voice box (larynx) at the entrance into the windpipe during swallowing, so that food and liquid do not enter the windpipe. Infants who have floppy cartilages that close prematurely when breathing and feeding can cause some pretty significant feeding problems and can affect the baby's ability to breath and swallow at the same time.

If your baby has this kind of noisy breathing, talk to your doctor, and discuss whether a referral to ENT is necessary.

There is a strong relationship between reflux and laryngomalacia. A study examined twenty-four children with laryngomalacia using a special pH (acid) monitoring device, and found that all (100 percent) had reflux

---

Severe Laryngomalacia or Something Else?

Go to the hospital immediately if your baby stops breathing for more than ten seconds, turns blue around the lips while breathing noisily, or pulls in at the neck or chest without relief after being repositioned or awakened.

---

into the throat. And anti-reflux treatment was associated with significant improvement of their breathing.[32] The diagnoses of respiratory reflux and of laryngomalacia can usually be made based upon a throat examination by a trained otolaryngologist. The exam is performed using an ultra-thin flexible camera (endoscope). With your infant awake, the ENT can safely pass this spaghetti-looking instrument (with a camera on its end) through your baby's nose and into the throat.

Most babies have a mild form of laryngomalacia, which does not interfere with feeding or sleeping. These infants can be expected to outgrow the noisy breathing by twelve to eighteen months of age, especially if reflux is controlled.

There exists, however, a small number of infants with laryngomalacia so severe that more drastic intervention is needed. These babies may take a long time to eat because it's hard for them to coordinate eating and breathing. They may also frequently turn "blue" or stop breathing, resulting in visits to the emergency room or hospitalization. Cases this severe must be referred to a pediatric ENT, as a full airway endoscopy under anesthesia is necessary, and often surgery may be recommended to clear the airway so that these babies can breathe more easily.

The procedure is relatively brief and it is performed endoscopically (through the mouth, leaving no scars on the neck) using either tiny, scissor-like instruments or a laser. This surgery typically works well and results in less noise and easier breathing. It also stops the blue spells, and since children who have the procedure breathe better, they will begin to feed better and gain weight.

Laryngospasm (Affects All Ages)

When reflux backs up from the esophagus and spills into the throat around the voice box, the vocal cords quickly clamp shut to protect against spillage into the lungs. This is part of the body's protective mechanism, trying to keep the lungs healthy from things that do not belong in them (like food, liquid, coins, other things that kids accidentally swallow). The larynx has receptors (like switches) that are triggered by acid and lead to sudden closure of the vocal cords. This is a little like getting a charley horse cramp in your calf: it will cause the muscles of the vocal folds to squeeze closed and will cause difficulty getting air into the lungs. This results in noisy breathing, especially during inhalation.[64]

Children of all ages as well as adults can have laryngospasm. Not every refluxer gets it, but some who frequently have respiratory reflux events may develop "trigger happy" vocal cords. Thankfully, most of the time, laryngospasm resolves spontaneously, within seconds to minutes, and even during the "attack," some air can get through.

Laryngospasm is one of the scariest events that a parent can experience, as it is obvious that their child is struggling to breathe, with a loud squeaking noise produced as air passes through an almost completely obstructed voice box. In infants with laryngospasm, they may temporarily stop moving altogether and grow limp. If this happens, parents need to attempt to stimulate the baby, call 911, and go to the emergency room.

In older children and adults, like in the case below, laryngospasm can occur at night, awakening a person from an otherwise sound sleep.

From the Case files of Dr. Julie: A Teenager with Laryngospasm

After midnight, a sixteen-year-old girl came running into her mother's room clutching her throat, gasping that she couldn't breathe. She passed out, and her mother called 911. When paramedics arrived, they emergently intubated her by placing a breathing tube through her voice box. She was then transferred to a children's hospital where she stayed in the intensive care unit. There, she was temporarily put into an induced coma with a ventilator supporting her breathing.

The ENT service was consulted, because the girl's doctors couldn't explain why this event had happened. When Dr. Julie met the mother, she asked her to describe the events of that evening. The mother relayed to her that the family had gone to a wedding, where they enjoyed fried chicken, mashed potatoes, corn, and desserts. When they left the wedding at almost midnight, they stopped to eat at Taco Bell. The teenager drank a large cup of soda alongside tacos and burritos with hot sauce. Everyone went to bed as soon as they got home, and not long after the patient had gone to bed, she came running into her mother's room. Severe acid reflux caused her to have laryngospasm!

On a healthier diet, she never experienced this terrifying complication of respiratory reflux again.

Brief Resolved Unexplained Event
(BRUE) (Affects Infants)

In medical literature, there is a condition called a Brief Resolved Unexplained Event. Until relatively recently, BRUE was termed ALTE, Apparent Life-Threatening Event, and the terms may be used interchangeably.[110]

What is BRUE? Some babies may experience a frightening episode where they stop breathing (apnea), change color (blue, pale, or red), and become limp. This type of an episode must get evaluated as an emergency, as other potential associated conditions such as heart problems, seizures, etc., need to be ruled out. It is believed that the most common causes of BRUE are respiratory reflux, lung infections, and seizures.

An Italian study reported that a third of the babies with BRUE had reflux; however, we believe that the actual percentage of reflux-caused BRUE may be much higher. If your child has any of the above-described episodes, call your child's doctor immediately and/or take your baby to the nearest emergency department.

Sudden Infant Death Syndrome
(SIDS) (Affects Infants)

While the cause or causes of SIDS remain unknown, there is some data relating this mortal condition to immaturity of the brain and respiratory reflux.[34] Under normal circumstances, when laryngospasm occurs, normal infants, children, and adults continue to breathe, albeit through a narrowed airway. The reflex drive to sustain breathing originates in brain control systems. In babies, that system may take several months to mature. Thus, it is possible that apnea (stoppage of breathing) may occur in response to laryngospasm triggered by reflux. Many years ago, this was shown in an animal model, namely, that in response to acid being placed in the larynx, apnea occurred in immature animals.[34,109]

We certainly do not want to scare parents, but if your infant has reflux, we believe that it should be controlled. The American Academy of Pediatric has additional specific recommendations to help prevent SIDS.[88]

Foreign Bodies in the Airway
(Usually Affects Toddlers)

Small children, especially toddlers, often put things in their mouths, including objects that they find on the floor. Most parents have a story of their baby eating their dog's food or perhaps a pretty marble. When small children swallow objects, like small plastic toy parts, for example, they may go down the wrong pipe and lodge in the airway, usually in the trachea or bronchial tubes. The most dangerous situation occurs when the object obstructs the airway and hinders breathing.

While foreign body ingestion usually occurs as an acute event—the baby was breathing fine and then suddenly there was a problem—this is not always the case, particularly if the foreign object is just small enough to move around the tracheobronchial tree (the large airway that connects the throat to the lungs). The reason this is relevant is that we have been discussing the role of reflux in chronic coughing and congestion. Having a foreign body lodged in the airway can lead to similar symptoms as well.

We have also discussed the possibility of chronic nasal congestion being a manifestation of reflux. In young children with a persistent one-sided discolored nasal discharge, it is important to rule-out the possibility of the child having a foreign body in the nasal passages. Your pediatrician should see your child if such an issue occurs.

The vocal cords are the most lethal place for a foreign body to get lodged. Hot dogs (of any size), uncut grapes, and hard candy can lodge at

---

From the Case Files of Dr. Julie: Bronchial Foreign Body

A three-year-old boy presented with intermittent wheezing and breathing problems that apparently started after he had been eating peanuts, six weeks prior. His parents took him to the emergency room shortly after the "event," and he was evaluated by examination and chest X-ray and discharged with the assumption that everything was fine. In the following weeks, however, he had intermittent noisy breathing, and sometimes, even gasped for air. He came to Dr. Julie and had a repeat chest X-ray that was normal. She recommended an examination under anesthesia; and sure enough Dr. Julie found a whole peanut in the left bronchus just below the area where the windpipe splits toward the right and left lungs. Removal of the peanut resolved the child's breathing problems.

the level of the vocal cords and completely block breathing, often with a disastrous outcome before even making it to the hospital. Peanuts are small and smooth enough to slip through the vocal cords, and may then cause airway obstruction or infection in the lung. Please, do not give these foods to young children, and follow the AAP recommendations for the various ages at which to introduce different foods. As a warning to parents, child-proof your home so that small consumable items, especially small plastic toys or parts of toys, are out of reach of your toddler.

While we are on the topic of foreign bodies that your child may consume, this point is *extremely* important: do *not* have button batteries lying around the house. Lithium batteries (button batteries) can be a life-threatening ingestion for your child. Damage from the injury caused by a button battery can be permanent and can affect the nasal passages, ears, food pipe, windpipe, and other major and vital structures in that area of the body. There is a two-hour window to remove the battery in case of ingestion, so please be vigilant if you suspect this has occurred!

Allergy and Asthma (Affects All Ages)

Allergies and asthma patients are frequently encountered in our practices. In fact, many of these children come to an ENT specialist before ever seeing an allergist or before having an allergy evaluation by their pediatrician. When we see a child who may have eczema, a family history of significant allergies, possible mold exposure at school or at home, vomiting after eating salmon, or difficulty breathing while playing outdoors (but no such issues indoors), we immediately suspect allergies. We recommend such children undergo an allergy evaluation to identify what may be triggering their symptoms, as opposed to simply prescribing allergy medications. Maybe simply avoiding a certain item in their diet or particular allergens at home or outside can help reduce the symptoms, and your child need not be on medicines that affect the entire body and brain.

In the ENT world, we think about hyperactivity during the daytime as being caused by sleep disturbance related to large tonsils and adenoids, but what if there is something your child is allergic to that is driving them off the wall? Studies have shown that children who are on allergy medications can exhibit some behavioral issues as well. But like in many other areas in medicine, there is no definitive research-based evidence that proves a causal relationship, and doctors have different opinions on this topic.

Often, healthy children with chronic cough, nasal stuffiness or congestion, and even "wheezing" are presumed to have allergies and/or asthma. They are prescribed nasal steroid sprays, oral antihistamines (which reduce allergy symptoms such as runny nose, congestion, itching of eyes, and sneezing), and even a medication called leukotriene receptor antagonist (LTRA), which relaxes the airways in the lungs to help prevent bronchospasm, or narrowing of the airway channels (an "asthma attack"). This medication helps to reduce the body's response to triggers that bring on allergy symptoms, including trees, grass, dust mites, pollen, mold, etc.

Acid reflux, however, can trigger the same reaction in the bronchioles and the lungs as in real asthma, causing the smooth muscles around the bronchioles to contract and tighten, making the channels for airflow narrower so that a person would appear to be having a harder time breathing in.

Both allergies and asthma can be "proven" by medical tests.[111,112] The most common items associated with food allergies in children are eggs, milk, and peanuts. Most children outgrow their allergies to milk and eggs, but often nut allergies remain. Children ages six months and older can be evaluated by receiving a skin prick test, also called a puncture or scratch test, which can check for immediate allergic reactions to as many as forty different substances at once.[112]

Another type of skin testing is intradermal, where potential triggers are injected into the skin. To check for food allergies in infants and young children, a pediatrician may order a blood test called RAST (radioallergosorbent) or ImmunoCAP, which measures the amount of allergen-specific immunoglobulin (IgE) antibody to specific food(s) being tested for or to particular environmental allergen exposures. In general, an allergist will take a thorough family history and review your child's condition in order to determine what to test for.

Allergy-like symptoms are often very difficult to pin down, because infants and young children can have runny noses and congestion for a variety of reasons: colds, teething, and often due to acid reflux causing excessive nasal symptoms.

To test if someone has asthma or other conditions that affect one's ability to breathe, pulmonary function tests (PFTs) may be performed. This is a group of tests that measure how well the lungs can take in and breathe out air, as well as how efficiently they transfer oxygen into the blood. Pulmonary function tests are also called spirometry or lung function tests. Most kids are able to perform these tests by six years of age, though some can do so at a younger age.[112,113] Children need to be old enough to follow directions and cooperate in order to complete these tests. Once again, acid reflux can cause bronchoconstriction, which can show up as "asthma" on the PFT, when in fact, without the acid reflux, the child may be able to breathe without difficulty or tightness.

Aspiration (Affects All Ages)

If food and liquid penetrates through the vocal cords and down the windpipe, doctors call it "aspiration." If, in the past, you have drunk water too quickly and started coughing/hacking as a result, then you are familiar with your body's typical response to feeling something go down the "wrong pipe."

Healthy babies, children, and adults are usually capable of coughing back out anything that accidentally gets into the windpipe, so they don't "aspirate" the substance into their lungs. Children who have underlying neurologic conditions, such as cerebral palsy, are at risk of having decreased ability to protect their airways while swallowing. These children are vulnerable to aspiration as a result of difficulty coordinating breathing and swallowing safely, a function we all take for granted.

The vocal cords are really pretty remarkable. When we breathe in, they open to create a triangular space for air to flow through into the windpipe and lungs. When we want to speak, they come together in a closed position, as air vibrates against their delicate folds to create sound.

The vocal cords and larynx (voice box) also protect our lungs from foreign objects like food, drinks, and inhaled particles. When this area of the voice box senses that something does not belong, it responds with a cough. This is called the laryngeal adductor reflux (LAR). It is a protective reflex that keeps our body safe and our lungs healthy.

In people who have significant reflux, it has been shown that the LAR is faulty, and sensation in the structures above the vocal cords may decrease. When water is swallowed (or worse, soda), there is decreased sensation of it coming down (or regurgitating up), and it can more easily travel down the "wrong pipe" (aspiration) into the lungs.

If this happens on a regular basis, your child may develop chronic problems like recurrent pneumonias or damage in the lungs. Some babies who choke each time they drink may end up needing a swallowing evaluation called a modified barium swallow (also known as a video swallow study), a type of X-ray study that looks at the flow of food and drink from the mouth to the stomach. Food should go straight into the food pipe and down into the stomach; if it slips into the trachea and lungs, that's a problem. Some babies get this type of aspiration from having bad reflux. Others may have structural problems that can lead to aspiration or functional issues like abnormal movement of their vocal cords due to neurological dysfunction in the brain.

Glottic and Subglottic Stenosis (Affect All Ages)

Glottic and subglottic stenoses describe a narrowing at the level of the vocal cords (glottis) and immediately below the vocal cords (subglottis). This is most commonly due to scarring or thick extra tissue obstructing airflow. In infants and children, the most common cause of scarring in these areas is prolonged intubation (breathing tube placed through the voice box) due to premature birth. Having a tube in the voice box for days, weeks, and even months can lead to reactive changes such as swelling, inflammation, and trauma to fragile tissue that lead to eventual scar formation.

Very rarely, children may require intubation for anesthesia for their procedures and surgery. Even if the intubation was just for a few hours, children may develop glottic and subglottic stenosis. Premature and young infants are especially vulnerable due to their very small airways. Without a history of intubation or any trauma to the voice box, the next most common reason for airway narrowing may be that a child is born with narrowing due to the shape of their cricoid cartilage. Reflux can cause inflammation in the airway and can also lead to swelling in a child's windpipe, worsening symptoms in those who may already have underlying structural airway abnormalities. Since reflux is very common in children, glottic and subglottic stenoses caused simply by reflux do occur.[20,24] Indeed, all cases of subglottic stenosis in children over one year of age should be considered reflux-related until proven otherwise.

Infants and children with narrowing in the glottis or subglottis usually produce noise while breathing in and out and may experience difficulty breathing. These symptoms are often made worse during viral illnesses. If your child has a history of requiring intubation and has developed noisy breathing both "in" and "out" and/or has labored breathing, talk to your child's doctor, and consider referral to an ENT specialist. Airway endoscopy can be performed under general anesthesia so that an ENT can see if there is any stenosis, narrowing, or swelling.

Bronchopulmonary Dysplasia (BPD) (Affects Infants)

Bronchopulmonary dysplasia (BPD) was first described by Northway and colleagues in 1967 as a lung injury in premature babies who needed intubation, mechanical ventilation (machine breathing for them), and oxygen support.[116] The more premature the baby is at the time of birth, the more the chance that their lungs are not ready and may require temporary intubation and mechanical ventilation. Specialists who help premature babies, called neonatologists, try to minimize the risk of BPD by giving surfactant.

Surfactant allows the lung alveolar sacs to remain open and reduces surface tension. Surfactant is delivered using an artificial airway or breathing tube that is inserted into the trachea, or windpipe, either immediately at birth for extremely premature babies or later, once there are signs of respiratory problems. It is extremely common for premature babies to have BPD, which is treated with a steroid through a nebulizer and other medications to keep the airways in the lungs open.

Premature infants and children also have a higher risk of acid reflux, due to their immature digestive systems and the tone of the lower esophageal sphincter. Research using pH impedance shows that infants with BPD are more prone to reflux.[114] Most premature infants do eventually outgrow BPD, but preventing reflux may help their lung function and prevent further damage. It is worth pointing out that there may be a relationship between respiratory reflux and bronchopulmonary dysplasia.[116] Further research is needed in this area.

Cystic Fibrosis

Cystic Fibrosis (CF) is a genetic condition that leads to chronic problems with the lungs and digestive system. It affects around 30,000 children and adults in the United States and about 70,000 worldwide.[117] Children who are born with CF have inherited a defective gene from each of their parents. This leads to the abnormal production of a very thick mucus that plugs the lungs, pancreas, and other organs. When this mucus plugs the lungs, it can cause breathing difficulties and can also be a source for infections. Think about how a puddle of standing water acts like a Petri dish for germs.

You may be wondering why three otolaryngologists are discussing CF. Patients with cystic fibrosis almost universally develop nasal polyps and difficulty with sinuses and nasal airway breathing. These nasal polyps can lead to chronic congestion in the nose that is then treated as chronic or recurrent sinus infections. CF can be associated with a chronic wet/phlegmy cough and with recurring pneumonias and other lung infections.

Once the sinuses are filled, some children develop headaches that can negatively impact their quality of life. Shortness of breath and asthma-like symptoms are frequently seen, and lack of weight gain can be a problem, too. As CF patients' noses and sinuses are naturally colonized by various bacteria, the pulmonologist (the primary specialist that cares for this group of patients) always wants to ensure that the sinuses are as healthy as possible in order to better protect the lungs.

Treatment for CF is quite extensive. Patients living with CF have daily routines to help them clear their mucous and stay healthy, involving a team of specialists with expertise in this field. Respiratory reflux has been shown to have a detrimental impact on the lungs of children with CF. Many CF patients do not make adequate digestive enzymes and may depend on external sources of those enzymes in the form of medications.

The exact frequency of reflux in CF patients is unknown, but the prevalence has been reported to be as high as 81 percent.[117] A study of twenty-five CF patients at Cincinnati Children's Hospital[119] looked at lung outcomes following surgical treatment of reflux (fundoplication; see page 174). In their study, the most common presenting symptoms of reflux were recurrent vomiting and poor weight gain. Significant improvement in pulmonary function was demonstrated after fundoplication.[120]

Gastrointestinal Problems

Constipation

If your child is chronically constipated, then stomach contents, including gastric juices and food/beverages, can regurgitate up through the esophagus and into the mouth. When this happens, your child may experience symptoms of respiratory reflux such as chronic coughing, congestion, croupy cough, nasal infections, ear infections, and more.

Constipation can be related to your baby's diet or to your toddler's desire to avoid the bathroom. Older children and teenagers can also experience chronic constipation. In these cases, a pediatrician or potentially a gastrointestinal specialist will likely need to intervene. A basic guide to help relieve constipation includes ensuring excellent hydration with regular water intake, increased fiber in the diet, spending a good amount of time on the toilet (try the step-stool to change the angle of the intestines), offering prune juice, and possibly laxatives. These methods should be done in concert with a consultation with your pediatrician. For more information on the frequency and health of bowel movements, see page 23 in Chapter 3.

Pyloric Stenosis

Pyloric stenosis is a condition that affects about three out of 1,000 babies in the United States, and it affects boys four times more frequently than girls. The reason for this gender bias is unknown. There are also reports that pyloric stenosis can run in families—meaning if a parent had pyloric stenosis there is up to twenty percent chance a baby may develop it.[84]

Pyloric stenosis is a condition in which the pylorus, a muscular valve between the stomach and small intestine, is too narrow, preventing food in the stomach from passing through and resulting in what's called "gastric outlet obstruction."

Most infants with pyloric stenosis develop symptoms about three-to-five weeks after birth. Because milk cannot empty from the stomach into the small intestine, babies with pyloric stenosis will have more than just spit up; they will have projectile vomiting. This is vomiting where formula is forcefully spit out of the mouth, even over a distance of several feet! Such vomiting can happen both soon after feeding or even hours later.

Babies with pyloric stenosis will vomit but soon want to feed again because they are not getting breast milk or formula into their intestines. Since they are not full or satiated, babies may also experience poor weight gain, poor growth, smaller stools, and/or constipation. If your baby has projectile vomiting, contact your pediatrician immediately.

Eosinophilic Esophagitis

Eosinophilic esophagitis (EoE) is a chronic allergic and immune condition. A child or adult with EoE will have chronic inflammation of the esophagus. Eosinophils are a type of white blood cell that is normally not found in the tissue of the esophagus; however, in EoE, large amounts of eosinophils migrate to the esophagus and cause "inflammation," as if responding to an allergic reaction triggered by food and/or something in the environment.

Different age groups may experience different symptoms of EoE. Infants and toddlers may not seem interested in eating or may refuse food to the point that their growth is inhibited due to inadequate nutrition. When the esophagus is inflamed, there is likely more reflux and pain, which leads to an eating aversion. Older, school-age children may complain of frequent belly aches and vomiting and claim that they can't swallow or have food stuck in their throat. Teenagers and adults will complain mostly of difficulty swallowing, especially dry and dense foods like bread and chicken.

One diagnostic symptom of EoE is a food impaction (like a piece of meat getting stuck in the food pipe). Chronic inflammation of the mucous membrane of the esophagus and the underlying muscles that contract to move food down the swallowing tube can cause narrowing (strictures) to the point that food just can't go down. Patients can feel this as a very uncomfortable pressure in their chest. If your child is having difficulty swallowing or is experiencing GI issues, consider talking to your pediatrician about EoE.

From the Case Files of Dr. Karen:
Eosinophilic Esophagitis

A twelve-year-old presented with a history of frequently recurring "colds," chronic cough, asthma, and sleep apnea. Allergy testing showed environmental allergies to trees, grass, pollen, dust mites, etc. Benadryl didn't help, nor did her asthma medications. The patient also had eczematous skin rashes, and dermatologic creams did little to alleviate her chronic itching and discomfort.

The patient was a competitive dancer. Her dietary habits included eating dinner at 6:00 p.m. or at 8:00 p.m., depending on her dance rehearsal schedule. Bedtime was usually around 9:30 p.m. Every night before bed, she would eat fruit. She also drank a lot of milk and loved ketchup and spicy food, even though eating spicy food would make her feel sick. Over time, the patient started to develop choking episodes with meats.

During her first the office visit, it was noted that she had a raspy voice and was frequently clearing her throat. A previous swallowing study had shown reflux. Given that her "asthma" was poorly controlled despite multiple medications, Dr. Karen performed an airway endoscopy with a GI colleague and diagnosed respiratory reflux and EoE.

She was treated with a strict reflux dietary program (see "A Twelve-Point Program for Healthier Eating," page 62), anti-reflux medications, and a swallowed steroid spray. Within six weeks, the patient's swallowing was normal, her voice no longer raspy, and her "asthma" cured.

In the past two decades, increased awareness has helped doctors[121] more successfully diagnose and treat EoE using dietary modifications, reflux medicine, and steroids.

Malrotation of the Bowel

If a child or an infant experiences vomiting with bile (green or yellow-brown intestinal fluid), they must be evaluated for a condition called malrotation/volvulus. Malrotation of the intestine is a surgical emergency. It means that the intestine (bowel) is improperly fixed in the abdominal cavity, leading it to twist and kink that prevents movement of stool. If not repaired in a timely fashion, this can lead to permanent damage to the intestines, dangerous infections, and even death.

Every child with bile vomiting should be evaluated for a malrotation with a swallowing study to confirm normal anatomy of the intestines. The treatment for malrotation of the intestines is surgical.[122]

Combined Gastrointestinal and Airway Problems

Recurrent Pneumonia

Getting pneumonia, particularly recurrent pneumonias, is not normal. While it can be a one-time event caused by a virus or bacteria, pneumonia may be a red flag for a congenital anatomic abnormality, a primary lung disease, or even a problem with the immune system. That said, severe reflux can cause recurrent pneumonia if a child has reflux into the lungs.

For most children that we see with recurrent pneumonia, the underlying mechanism is aspiration: liquid and/or stomach contents going "down the wrong pipe." For this reason, children with recurrent pneumonias must be medically evaluated, and underlying problems must be ruled out. Your doctor may suggest diagnostic testing, possibly including a chest X-ray, swallowing evaluations, office-based endoscopy, or even an examination under anesthesia.

Tracheoesophageal Fistula and Esophageal Atresia

Under normal circumstances, there is a shared, common anatomic wall between the trachea (breathing tube) and the esophagus (swallowing tube). The esophagus is situated behind the trachea. If there is a hole in

From the Case Files of Dr. Karen:
Tracheoesophageal Fistula

A three-year-old boy was born with a condition called tracheoesophageal fistula (TEF). This is a condition in which a baby has an abnormal connection between the windpipe (trachea) and swallowing tube (esophagus). This condition was quickly diagnosed after birth, because every time the baby fed, he would turn blue along with coughing, gagging, and difficulty breathing as milk entered the windpipe from the esophagus, soiling the lungs. The baby's breathing sounded like a "washing machine." The neonatologist (a doctor that takes care of newborn babies) ordered a barium swallow X-ray that showed spilling of the barium (the contrast material) into the trachea from the esophagus. (This constant spillage of food into the lungs (aspiration) can result in pneumonia and lung damage.) A pediatric surgeon was consulted who repaired the TEF by closing the connection between the windpipe and esophagus.

Over time, the baby continued to have some noisy breathing on and off as well as reflux; however, dietary modifications and a low-acid diet were sufficient to effectively treat the baby's lingering symptoms.

this wall, aspiration will occur with all feeding. This can manifest as coughing, wheezing, turning blue with feeding, and recurring pneumonias. Such openings are called tracheoesophageal fistulas, or TEF. The TEF may be associated with an esophageal atresia (EA), which is a congenital defect occurring in about one per 4,000 babies. In most cases of esophageal atresia, the upper esophagus ends in a blind pouch and is not connected with the lower part of the esophagus or stomach. Other configurations of EA/TEF abnormalities are possible.

Most infants with EA not only have two separate parts of the esophagus that do not connect to one another, they also usually have a TEF in which there is a pathologic connection between the trachea and the esophagus. In addition, infants with EA/TEF often have a "floppy" or weak trachea, called tracheomalacia. Having tracheomalacia can cause a baby to have noisy or high-pitched breathing due to excessive movement and floppiness of the trachea during breathing. This noise can sound like a washing machine. Almost fifty percent of babies born with EA and TEF also have other birth defects.

Children and babies with a EA/TEF, and also those in post repair of this condition, can have pooling of secretions in the voice box, which can lead to voice and airway problems. Too much pooling of salivary secretions (or mucous) because of difficulty swallowing or too much reflux because of a floppy esophagus can lead to reflux symptoms that you are by now familiar with. For more information, you can look up the EA/TEF child and family support webpage at http://www.eatef.org.[123]

Congenital Diaphragmatic Hernia

The diaphragm is a thin muscular barrier that normally separates the chest cavity from the abdomen. It also functions as a bellows that is vital to breathing. When the diaphragm contracts downward, the lungs fill with air (inspiration), and when it contracts upward, the air in the lungs is emptied (expiration). The esophagus normally resides above the diaphragm and the stomach below. Normally, there is a small opening in the diaphragm through which the esophagus passes.

Congenital diaphragmatic hernia is a condition in which this opening is greatly oversized, allowing the stomach to ride up into the chest. Depending on the size of this hernia, the entire stomach can end up in the chest cavity, and the space it occupies can compromise breathing, as the volume of the lungs is reduced by the mass effect of the stomach. Compromised breathing is manifest from birth. This condition requires diagnosis by X-ray and surgical correction.[124]

Cricopharyngeal Achalasia

The cricopharyngeus (CP) muscle is located behind the voice box, at the entrance to the esophagus. It is the upper gatekeeper to the esophagus, and when it relaxes, it allows food and liquids to enter the food pipe. When it is tight, it prevents air from being swallowed during breathing. These are its basic functions. If the CP muscle is too tight and does not properly relax, it is referred to as CP achalasia (failure to relax). When a child has CP achalasia, symptoms can include regurgitation into the nasal passages, choking spells, swallowing difficulty, aspiration, and weight loss.

Sometimes, a baby may present significant projectile vomit through the nose as another clinical sign. Reflux is very commonly associated and can sometimes be confused with CP achalasia. In order to diagnose this condition, a video swallowing study (a.k.a. a modified barium swallow) needs to be done, during which a radiologist will notice a finding called the CP Bar, a spasm of the CP muscle when it fails to relax during swallowing. While CP achalasia is rare, a physician should have a high index of suspicion in children because it requires a radiologist to look for it, and it is, therefore, easily missed. Currently, the treatment modality in children is varied. Some report benefits from a Botox injection into the muscle, dilation (stretching) of the muscle, or surgery.[125]

Cardiac and Neurological Problems

Medical conditions related to circulation in the body and muscle tone can both worsen and mimic symptoms of reflux. Difficulty or turning blue with feeding, noisy or labored breathing, reflux-type symptoms, congestion, sleep apnea, laryngomalacia, and many of the topics we have covered in this book can be associated with heart (cardiac) and neurological conditions.

Reflux has been reported to occur in as many as seventy percent of patients with neurological impairment.[126] In such patients, adjusting diet, thickening of meals to reduce possible regurgitation, placement on anti-reflux medications, and sometimes performing surgery can help control symptoms and avoid the complications of reflux. It is beyond the scope of this book to cover these topics in detail, but it is important to understand that they exist. Again, consult your pediatrician if your child presents symptoms that worry you.

How to Read a Nutrition Label

Before revealing the nuts and bolts behind the somewhat confusing nutritional fact label, we need to emphasize that you must look at the ingredients, especially for items that are staples in your house, the things you buy every week. If you cook with store-bought chicken or vegetable stock, for example, pick a brand that does not have sugar added (most do). Likewise, look at the sugar and fat content. If the first ingredient is sugar (see below), beware. The same is true of fat, not to mention unpronounceable chemicals.

Sugar by Any Other Name Would Still Be Sugar

There are many names for various types of added sugar, so when you are reading the ingredient list, please beware that processed foods may contain up to 74 percent added sugar! Unless you are familiar with the many names of sugar you may not realize how much added sugar is in the foods and beverages you buy. Common names may include sucrose, high-fructose corn syrup, dextrose, maltose, and rice syrup.[12,127,128]

When reading the nutrition fact label, pay attention to the *total* sugar, *natural* sugar, and *added* sugar. Natural sugars include those found in fruits and vegetables, such as fructose, and some found in dairy, such as lactose. Added sugars provide little or no nutritional value. Avoid products with sugar listed as one of the first three ingredients, since ingredients that weigh the most are listed first.

The Aliases of Sugar

Agave nectar
Barbados sugar
Barley malt
Barley malt syrup
Beet sugar
Brown sugar
Buttered syrup
Cane juice
Cane juice crystals
Cane sugar
Caramel
Carob syrup
Castor sugar
Coconut palm sugar
Coconut sugar
Confectioner's sugar
Corn sweetener
Corn syrup
Corn syrup solids
Date sugar
Dehydrated cane juice
Demerara sugar
Dextrin
Dextrose
Evaporated cane juice
Free-flowing brown sugars
Fructose
Fruit juice
Fruit juice concentrate
Glucose
Glucose solids

Golden sugar
Golden syrup
Grape sugar
HFCS (High-Fructose
    Corn Syrup)
Honey
Icing sugar
Invert sugar
Malt syrup
Maltodextrin
Maltol
Maltose
Mannose
Maple syrup
Molasses
Muscovado
Palm sugar
Panocha
Powdered sugar
Raw sugar
Refiner's syrup
Rice syrup
Saccharose
Sorghum Syrup
Sucrose
Sugar (granulated)
Sweet Sorghum
Syrup
Treacle
Turbinado sugar
Yellow sugar

Fats

There are two main groups of fats, the "good" fat or unsaturated fat, versus the "bad" fat also known as saturated fat. Basically, eat as much good fat as possible and avoid "trans fat" as much as possible. In general, products containing fat that is twenty percent or higher of the daily percentage value is considered high and bad for health.

The Bad Fats

Saturated animal fat

Bacon
Butter
Cheese
Cream cheese
Ice cream
Lard
Whole milk

Plant-based fats that have been hydrogenated contain trans fats.

Biscuits
Breakfast sandwiches
Cakes, pies, cookies
Fried foods
Frosting
Frozen pizza
Margarines
Processed baked goods (dough nuts, muffins, etc.)
Shortenings

The Good Fats

Unsaturated or good fats include polyunsaturated fats, which are found mostly in vegetable oils, including:

Corn oil
Fish, such as salmon, mackerel, herring, albacore tuna, and trout
Flax seeds or flax oil
Safflower oil
Soybean oil
Sunflower seeds
Walnuts

Monounsaturated fats also can help lower cholesterol, triglycerides, and improve heart health. These include:

Avocado	Safflower oil (high oleic)
Canola oil	Sesame oil
Olive oil	Sunflower oil
Peanut oil and butter.	

Everyone knows about the omega-3s that are found in fatty fish, such as salmon, trout, mackerel, flaxseeds and walnuts

There are two types of trans fats, naturally occurring in dairy and meat, and the more common artificial trans fat found when liquid oils are hardened into "partially hydrogenated fats." This is the stuff used in frying, baked goods, doughnuts, margarine, cookies, icing, crackers, processed snacks, microwave popcorn—you know, all the stuff we all *love* because it tastes *so good!*

Every child deserves some cupcake, cake, cookies, doughnuts, and other sweet treats for special occasions or as a treat, but try to avoid eating such foods on a daily basis. Daily consumption of trans fats along with sugar will surely result in gaining of excessive weight and risk of obesity.

NUTRITION FACTS LABEL

Reading and understanding the nutrition facts label on prepared foods can be challenging, even for savvy shoppers. However, the information listed below can help you make healthier choices when shopping.

Each label includes details about:

›› **What is in the product**   ›› **What the size of each serving is**   ›› **How much you are getting per serving**

SERVINGS PER CONTAINER

Tells you *how many* servings are included in the entire container.

SERVINGS SIZE

Tells you how much is considered 1 serving. The facts listed are all based on 1 serving.

PERCENT DAILY VALUE

Tells you what percentage of your total recommended daily intake is contained in this item.

CALORIES

Remember that this is per serving. So if you ate the entire container, that's 8 servings and you consumed 230 x 8 or 1,840 calories!

The left column lists TOTAL amounts for calories, fat, cholesterol, sodium, carbohydrates, and protein, per single serving.

CARBOHYDRATE

Includes sugar, sugar alcohol, starches, and fiber.

TIP Choose items higher in fiber, ideally more than 3 grams of fiber per serving.

Nutrition Facts

8 servings per container
Serving size   2/3 cup (55g)

Amount per serving
Calories   230

	% Daily Value*
Total Fat 8g	**10%**
Saturated Fat 1g	**5%**
Trans Fat 0g	
Cholesterol 0mg	**0%**
Sodium 160mg	**7%**
Total Carbohydrate 37g	**13%**
Dietary Fiber 4g	**14%**
Total Sugars 12g	
Includes 10g Added Sugars	**20%**
Protein 3g	
Vitamin D 2mcg	10%
Calcium 260mg	20%
Iron 8mg	45%
Potassium 235mg	6%

* The % Daily Value (DV) tells you how much a nutrient in a serving of food contributes to a daily diet. 2,000 calories a day is used for general nutrition advice.

TOTAL FAT   0g FAT FREE

The total amount of fat per serving of this product.

SATURATED FAT

Try to eat as little saturated fat as possible. Avoid trans fat.

TOTAL SUGARS

Tells you how much sugar is in the item per serving, including both natural and added. Added sugar in the next line tells you what was added during processing or production.

MICRONUTRIENTS

These are listed at the bottom of the label. The ones required to be listed by law are Iron, Calcium, Vitamin D and Potassium, since these are often deficient in American diets. They are important for children's growth and development.

INGREDIENT LIST

The ingredient list is usually located below the nutrition facts label.

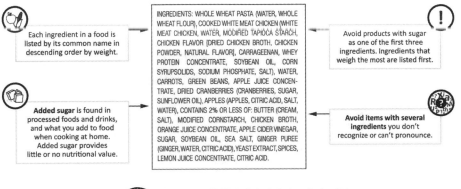

Each ingredient in a food is listed by its common name in descending order by weight.

Avoid products with sugar as one of the first three ingredients. Ingredients that weigh the most are listed first.

INGREDIENTS: WHOLE WHEAT PASTA (WATER, WHOLE WHEAT FLOUR), COOKED WHITE MEAT CHICKEN (WHITE MEAT CHICKEN, WATER, MODIFIED TAPIOCA STARCH, CHICKEN FLAVOR [DRIED CHICKEN BROTH, CHICKEN POWDER, NATURAL FLAVOR], CARRAGEENAN, WHEY PROTEIN CONCENTRATE, SOYBEAN OIL, CORN SYRUPSOLIDS, SODIUM PHOSPHATE, SALT), WATER, CARROTS, GREEN BEANS, APPLE JUICE CONCENTRATE, DRIED CRANBERRIES (CRANBERRIES, SUGAR, SUNFLOWER OIL), APPLES (APPLES, CITRIC ACID, SALT, WATER), CONTAINS 2% OR LESS OF: BUTTER (CREAM, SALT), MODIFIED CORNSTARCH, CHICKEN BROTH, ORANGE JUICE CONCENTRATE, APPLE CIDER VINEGAR, SUGAR, SOYBEAN OIL, SEA SALT, GINGER PUREE (GINGER, WATER, CITRIC ACID), YEAST EXTRACT, SPICES, LEMON JUICE CONCENTRATE, CITRIC ACID.

Added sugar is found in processed foods and drinks, and what you add to food when cooking at home. Added sugar provides little or no nutritional value.

Avoid items with several ingredients you don't recognize or can't pronounce.

TIP

Use the ingredient list to find out whether a food or drink contains ingredients that are sources of nutrients you want more of (e.g., contain whole grains) or sources of nutrients you want less of (e.g., partially hydrogenated oils contain trans fat and corn syrup solids are an added sugar).

IMPORTANT THINGS TO REMEMBER

» **Sugar comes in many forms.** It can be listed as powdered sugar, dextrose, high fructose corn syrup, maple sugar, rice syrup, cane juice, and many more.

» **Every four grams of sugar is equivalent to about one teaspoon of sugar.** If a serving contains 12 grams of sugar that's three teaspoons of sugar.

» **A 12-fluid ounce can of soda has about 40 to 50 grams of added sugar,** so it can contain 10–12 teaspoons of sugar!

» **Natural sugar** is found in whole, unprocessed foods such as fruits, vegetables, some grains and dairy. Fruits contain the natural sugar fructose, while lactose is a natural sugar found in dairy products.

» **For fat, generally 5% is considered low and 20% is considered high.** The quality of fats differs but, as a general rule, try to eat as little saturated fat as possible and avoid trans fat altogether.

» **Just because the label only states a few micronutrients,** this does not mean that other vitamins and minerals are not present in this item. Vitamin D and Potassium are now required on labels because they are nutrients that Americans don't always get enough of and when lacking, are associated with increased risk of chronic disease.

Healthy Shopping Guide
and Meal Planning

When you go to the grocery store, be aware of the good, the bad, and what's best to leave out of your cart! Remember: you want to try and eat lean, clean, green, and alkaline (pages 68–70). Generally avoid buying processed meats, juice, soda, other soft drinks, too much dairy and junk food. Recommended for each person in your family is four to five servings of fruit and vegetables per day.

The pH (Acidity) Listing of Common Foods and Beverages

* Indicates more acidic than recommended; ** Indicates an item that may or may not be too acidic, but that is still not good for reflux for another reason. See also the baby food pH measurements on pages 29–30. (Note: some * foods may be consumed in moderation once reflux is controlled.)

Food or Drink	pH
Agave Nectar (Sweet Cactus Farms)	4.5
Almond Milk	6.5
Apples—Fiji	4.8
Apples—Gala	4.2*
Apples—Granny Smith	3.6*
Apples—Macintosh	3.7*
Apples—Macoun	3.2*
Apples—Red Delicious	4.5
Applesauce (Mott's Original)	3.4*
Avocado	7.8
Banana	5.6
Barbecue Sauce (Bull's-Eye Original)	3.7*
Barbecue Sauce (Kraft Original)	3.4*
Beets (Red)	6.1

Food or Drink	pH
Bell Pepper – Italian Stuffing Pepper	5.0
Bell Pepper (Green)	5.1
Bell Pepper (Orange)	4.8
Bell Pepper (Red)	4.9
Blackberries	3.7*
Blueberries	3.7*
Bottled Water (most)	7.0
Broccoli	6.3
Cabbage (Green)	6.0
Cabbage (Red)	6.3
Cabbage (Savoy)	6.1
Caesar Dressing (Newman's Own)	3.5*
Carrots	7.0
Cherries	3.9*
Coca-Cola Diet	3.7*
Coca-Cola	2.8*
Coffee (Strong Black)—limit one cup per day	5.0
Coffee (With Milk)—limit one cup per day	6.2
Coke Zero	3.3*
Corn	6.9
Cranberry Juice (Tropicana)	2.9*
Cranberry pomegranate Juice (Knudsen)	3.7*
Cream Soda (Dr. Brown's Diet)	4.5**
Cucumber	6.0
Diced Tomatoes (canned)	4.0*
Eggplant	6.0
Endive	6.0
Fennel	6.9
Gatorade (Fruit Punch)	3.0*
Ginger	6.5
Grape (Green, Seedless)	3.6*
Grapefruit (Pink)	3.4*
Green Beans – Canned, Cut (Green Giant)	5.2
Green beans	6.3
Hot Sauce (Texas Pete)	3.1*
Iced Tea (Lipton Lemon, bottled)	3.2*
Italian dressing (Zesty Kraft)	5.2
Ketchup (Heinz)	3.4*

Food or Drink	pH
Kiwi	3.4*
Lemon	2.9*
Lime	2.7*
Mandarin Oranges (Dole)	3.2*
Mango (Del Monte)	3.4*
Mango	3.7*
Melon (Ripe Cantaloupe)	6.1
Milk—Almond	6.5
Milk—Whole Processed cow	6.5**
Milk (2% Organic)	7.5
Milk (Lactaid Fat-Free)	7.0
Mountain Dew Diet	3.1*
Mushrooms (Domestic)	6.1
Mushrooms (Portobello)	6.5
Mustard (Dijon, Grey Poupon)	3.6*
Mustard (Yellow, White Rose)	3.2*
Nectarines	3.3*
Oatmeal with 2% Milk	7.2
Olives—Black, Pitted (Best Brand)	7.3
Onion (White)	6.0
Onions (Spanish Yellow Raw, White Sauté)	6.3**
Orange (Navel)	3.8*
Orange Juice	3.8*
Pancake Batter (Banana/Oatmeal)	6.8
Parsley—Italian Flat Leaf	6.1
Parsnip	6.6
Peaches	3.6*
Pear (Bosc)	5.3
Peas—Canned, Small (Le Sueur)	5.8
Pellegrino (and most brands of seltzer)	4.8**
Pepsi Diet	2.9*
Pepsi	3.5*
Pickle—Crunchy, Dill (B&G)	3.7*
Pineapple	3.4*
Pomegranate Cranberry Juice (Langer's)	2.8*
Pomegranate	3.3*
Potato (Idaho)	5.7
Potato (Yukon Gold)	6.0

Food or Drink	pH
Radish (Red or Black)	6.1
Ranch Dressing—Reduced Fat (Kraft)	3.9*
Raspberries	4.2*
Russian Dressing (Wishbone)	3.8*
Salsa—Mild Chunky (Tostitos)	3.7*
Seltzer (Seagram's Original)	3.8*
Snapple Diet Lemon	3.3*
Sparkling Water (Poland Spring)	4.3*
Sprite Zero	3.6*
Squash—Acorn	5.9
Squash—Spaghetti	6.2
Strawberries	3.5*
Tab Diet Soda	2.9*
Tap Water (New York City)	7.0
Tea (Lipton)	5.8
Tea (chamomile)	6.2
Tea (Chinese White Jasmine)	5.6
Thousand Island Dressing	3.6*
Tomato Juice (Campbell's From Concentrate)	3.9*
Tomato Paste (Hunt)	4.0*
Tomato Sauce (Del Monte)	3.9*
Tomatoes—Roma (Raw or Cooked)	4.4*
Tomatoes—Whole Peeled (San Marzano)	4.2*
Turnip	6.2
Worcestershire Sauce (Lea & Perrins)	3.4*
Yam	6.1
Yogurt—1% Peach	4.0*
Yogurt—Peach, Fruit on Bottom (Dannon)	4.5
Yogurt 1% Plain Milk Fat (Cream-O-Land)	4.3*
Zucchini	6.6

Recommended Books, Articles, Web Links, and Community Resources

Books

Campbell TC, Campbell TM II. *The China Study: Revised and Expanded Edition: The Most Comprehensive Study of Nutrition Ever Conducted and the Startling Implications for Diet, Weight Loss, and Long-Term Health.* Revised ed. Dallas: BenBella Books; 2016.

Davis, W. *Wheat Belly.* New York: Rodale; 2011.

Koufman J. *The Chronic Cough Enigma: How to Recognize, Diagnose and Treat Neurogenic and Reflux-Related Cough.* New York: Katalitix Media; 2014.

Koufman J, Huang S, Gelb P. *Dr. Koufman's Acid Reflux Diet: With 111 All New Recipes Including Vegan & Gluten-Free: The Never-Need-to-Diet-Again Diet.* Katalitix Media, New York; 2015.

Koufman J, Stern J, Bauer M. *Dropping Acid: The Reflux Diet Cookbook & Cure.* New York: The Reflux Cookbooks; 2010.

Lustig, R. *Fat Chance: Beating the Odds Against Sugar, Processed Food, Obesity, and Disease.* New York: Plume; 2013.

Moss M. *Salt, Sugar, Fat.* New York: Random House; 2013.

Perlmutter D, Loberg C. *Grain Brain: The Surprising Truth about Wheat, Carbs, and Sugar—Your Brain's Silent Killers.* New York: Little, Brown and Company; 2013.

Pollan M. *The Omnivore's Dilemma: A Natural History of Four Meals.* New York: Penguin; 2007.

Salatin J. *Folks, This Ain't Normal: A Farmer's Advice for Happier Hens, Healthier People, and a Better World.* Nashville: Center Street; 2012.

Wei J: *A Healthier Wei: Reclaiming Health for Misdiagnosed and Overmedicated Children.* New York: A Healthier Wei LLC; 2012.

Movies and Documentaries About the Food We Consume

Fed Up (on Netflix and Amazon)

Food, Inc. (on Netflix and Amazon)

Forks Over Knives (on Netflix and Amazon)

Wei J. TEDx *Talk: Milk and Cookie Disease.* Available at:
https://www.youtube.com/watch?v=R2C6bBNWGp0

What the Health (on Netflix)

Articles—Media

Koufman J. Obama's Acid Reflux May Help Others Receive Proper Diagnosis and Treatment. *Washington Post.* December 8, 2014.

Koufman J. The Dangers of Eating Late at Night. *New York Times.* October 25, 2014.

Koufman J. The Specialists' Stranglehold on Medicine. *New York Times.* June 3, 2017.

Generally Recognized as Safe (GRAS) List. Food Additive Status List. February 16, 2014.
http://www.fda.gov/Food/IngredientsPackagingLabeling/FoodAdditives
Ingredients/ucm091048.htm

Food Safety: FDA Should Strengthen Its Oversight of Food Ingredients Determined to Be Generally Recognized as Safe (GRAS).
http://www.gao.gov/products/GAO-10-246.

GAO-10-246: United States Government Accountability Office. February 3, 2010.

Articles—Scientific

Catassi C, Elli L, Bonaz B, et al. Diagnosis of non-celiac gluten sensitivity (ncgs): The salerno experts' criteria. *Nutrients 7.* 2015; 4966–77.

Hadjivassiliou M, Davies-Jones G, Sanders D, Grunewald R. Dietary treatment of gluten ataxia. *J Neurol Neurosurg Psychiatry.* 2003; 74:1221–24.

Hvid-Jensen F, Pedersen L, Funch-Jensen P, Drewes AM. Proton pump inhibitor use may not prevent high-grade dysplasia and oesophageal adeno-carcinoma in Barrett's oesophagus: a nationwide study of 9883 patients. *Alimentary Pharmacology and Therapeutics*. 2014; 1–8.

Johnston N, Dettmar PW, Bishwokarma B, Lively MO, Koufman JA. Activity/stability of human pepsin: implications for reflux attributed laryngeal disease. *Laryngoscope*. 2007;117:1036–9.

Shah NH, LePendu P, Bauer-Mehren A, et al. Proton pump inhibitor usage and the risk of myocardial infarction in the general population. *PLOS ONE*. 2015; 015 Jun 10;10(6):e0124653. doi: 10.1371/journal.pone.0124653. eCollection.

Weblinks

The Voice Institute of New York http://www.voiceinstituteofnewyork.com

Koufman J. Transnasal Esophagoscopy http://transnasalesophagoscopy.com

The Reflux Cookbook Blog http://www.refluxcookbookblog.com

American Academy of Pediatrics Juice Guidelines, go to American Academy of Pediatrics Infant Food and Feeding
https://www.aap.org/en-us/advocacy-and-policy/aap-health-initiatives/HALF-Implementation-Guide/Age-Specific-Content/pages/infant-food-and-feeding.aspx

American Academy of Pediatric Toddler Food and Feeding
https://www.aap.org/en-us/advocacy-and-policy/aap-health-initiatives/HALF-Implementation-Guide/Age-Specific-Content/Pages/Toddler-Food-and-Feeding.aspx

Children's books that teach healthy eating
https://www.weareteachers.com/11-fantastically-fun-childrens-books-that-teach-healthy-eating-habits

Community Resources

Center for Pediatric Airway Disorders, Children's Hospital of Philadelphia
http://www.chop.edu/centers-programs/center-pediatric-airway-disorders

Exercise and Eating Healthy Games for Kids
https://www.usa.gov/education?source=kids

National Early Care Education Learning Collaborative (ECELC)
https://healthykidshealthyfuture.org/about-ecelc/national-project

YMCA Healthy Eating Physical Activity, go to: http://www.ymca.net/hepa

Glossary

Acid reflux. A lay term for symptoms/disease caused by the backflow of gastric (stomach) contents upward into the *esophagus* (swallowing tube from the throat to the stomach) and airway (sinuses, nose, throat, mouth, breathing passages, and lungs). The most common symptoms of acid reflux are heartburn, indigestion, hoarseness, and cough.

Acid. Containing hydrogen ions, pH <7; see *pH scale*, page 4. The acidity of stomach acid is pH 2–4, and the same can be said of almost every soft drink, with ascorbic, citric, and phosphoric acid being the most commonly used preservatives.

Acid-suppressive, acid-suppression. This refers to decreasing the amount of acid that is produced by the stomach, specifically reducing the amount of acid produced by the acid secreting cells.

Acid-suppressive medications. Acid-suppressive (stomach-acid-reducing) medications generally fall into two classes, *proton pump inhibitors* (PPIs) and *H2-antagonists* (H2As). The PPIs (including Prilosec, Nexium, Dexilant, Prevacid, Protonix, Aciphex) are stronger and associated with rebound hyperacidity when stopped. The H2As (including Tagamet, Pepcid, and Zantac or ranitidine) have fewer side effects, work better at night, and are generally preferred to PPIs as over-the-counter anti-reflux medications. See *Proton pump inhibitor* and *H2-Antagonist* for more information.

Aerodigestive tract, aerodigestive. The *airway* and digestive tracts treated as one anatomical and functional system. The *digestive tract* starts at the mouth and ends at the anus; it includes the throat, esophagus, stomach, and intestines. See also *integrated aerodigestive medicine*.

Airway reflux testing. Reflux testing for the detection of airway reflux; see *pH monitoring*.

Airway. The breathing passages, from the tip of the nose to the root of the lungs. The airway includes the nose, throat, voice box (larynx), trachea, bronchi, and lungs.

Airway reflux. The backflow (reflux) of stomach contents into the airway, respiratory reflux. *Respiratory reflux* is also sometimes called *airway reflux, laryngopharyngeal reflux* (LPR), or *extraesophageal reflux*. *Respiratory reflux* causes many throat, sinus, and lung diseases and may be confused with other conditions such *asthma, allergies,* and *sinusitis.*

Albuterol. Albuterol is a medication that is usually used to treat asthma. It works by dilating (opening) the bronchial tubes; thus, it is a bronchodilator-type medication.

Alkaline water. Water that has a pH-value of more than 7 is technically alkaline; drinking water pH >8 is a useful adjunctive treatment for airway reflux, because *pepsin* is denatured (dies) at pH>8.

Alkaline. Not acidic, pH >7; see *pH scale.*

Allergists. Doctors who specialize in the diagnosis and treatment of allergies and allergic conditions.

Allergy. Abnormal reaction of the body to a previously encountered allergen, introduced by inhalation, ingestion, injection, or skin contact, often manifested by itchy eyes, runny nose, wheezing, skin rash, or diarrhea; a hypersensitivity reaction.

Anti-reflux medication (medical treatment). Such includes antacids (such as Tums, Rolaids, Gaviscon) as well as H2-antagonists and proton-pump inhibitors.

Anti-reflux surgery. This is a type of surgery that is used to treat reflux. The most effective and popular procedure is *lap fundoplication*, in which the dome of the stomach is loosened up and then wrapped around the esophagus and sewn there to create a tight angle so that what goes into the stomach stays in the stomach. This surgery is the best treatment we have; that is, it is even better than any medication. Surgery of this type is reserved for special cases since most reflux can be cured by healthy dietary and lifestyle changes.

Aspiration. Aspiration occurs when food or liquid is inhaled, spilled, or swallowed into the interior of the voice box and/or into the bronchi and lungs. Laymen refer to this as something "going down the wrong pipe." Aspiration usually causes intense and violent cough and can lead to pneumonia. Aspiration is one of the symptoms that people call "choking."

Asthma. Form of *reactive airway disease* characterized by constriction of the bronchi (the large airway tubes between the lower throat and the lungs); asthma is associated with difficulty getting air out (exhalation) and this type of airway obstruction (only during expiration) is called *wheezing*.

Barium swallow esophagogram. This is a video X-ray study of the swallowing mechanism. By swallowing a radio-opaque substance, barium, the entire tube of the throat and esophagus may be seen in real time. The barium swallow is not considered a good diagnostic for reflux; its main use is to examine for structural changes, e.g., cancer, diverticulum.

Bronchial, bronchus, bronchi. Referring to the bronchi, which are the two main breathing tubes and their branch points inside the lungs.

Bronchodilators. Type of medicine used to open up the bronchi when they are narrowed during an asthma attack, or for other reactive airways disorders.

Bronchoscopy. *Endoscopy* (internal examination) of the lungs, usually performed by a *pulmonologist*.

Choking, choking episodes. There are three different symptoms that people call choking: (1) If food or pills get stuck in the throat or esophagus, the choking is often related to narrowing of the esophagus due to *esophageal reflux*. (2) Inability to get air in during inhalation, usually due to *laryngospasm*, which is also usually caused by *airway reflux*. (3) Finally, choking occurs when food or drink "goes down the wrong pipe" into the trachea and lungs. This is called *aspiration*, and it can be a complication of *vocal cord paralysis* or *glottal insufficiency,*

Chronic bronchitis. Bronchitis (acute and chronic) is one of the most common causes of chronic cough and results from inflammation and infection in the airways of the lung. Bronchitis may be due to viral, bacterial, or fungal infection, or it may be a consequence of airway reflux.

Chronic cough. Defined as cough lasting more than eight weeks.

Cricoid cartilage. Signet-ring-shaped cartilage that sits immediately below the vocal cords and leads to the windpipe (trachea). The cricoid cartilage forms the foundation of the voice box and vocal cords.

Cricopharyngeal achalasia. Failure of the cricopharyngeus muscle to relax, causing a spasm in the upper esophagus that can affect swallowing.

Cricopharyngeal muscle. This is the muscle sphincter (also referred to as the upper esophageal sphincter) that sits at the upper part of the esophagus just behind and below the larynx. The terms cricopharyngeus and upper esophageal sphincter are used synonymously.

Digestive tract. All parts of the body involved in eating, swallowing, and digesting nutrients, including the mouth, tongue, throat, *esophagus, duodenum,* small intestine (jejunum and ileum), large bowel (colon), and rectum.

Duodenum. Uppermost part of the small intestine that is connected to the stomach and small bowel (jejunum) below; the gall bladder and pancreas drain into the duodenum.

Dysfunction. Malfunctioning, as of an organ or structure of the body.

Dysphagia. Difficulty swallowing.

Dysphonia. Hoarseness.

ENT (ear, nose, and throat) physician. Surgical specialist in diseases of the ears, nose, and throat; the specialty is called *otorhinolaryngology* or *otolaryngology—head and neck surgery.*

Erosive esophagitis. Reflux-related esophageal damage causing ulceration to the lining membrane (mucosa) in the area above the stomach. This diagnosis requires esophagoscopy and biopsy and is a complication of esophageal reflux, aka *GERD, gastroesophageal reflux disease.*

Esophageal atresia. An absence of part of the esophagus (food pipe) that occurs prior to birth and causes the baby to be born without a continuous passage for food from the throat to the stomach.

Esophageal reflux. Backflow of *gastric* (stomach) contents into the *esophagus.*

Esophageal spasm. One of the causes of reflux-caused chest pain, even crushing chest pain that can mimic a heart attack.

Esophageal stricture. With prolonged chronic or *chronic-intermittent* gastroesophageal reflux disease, the esophagus can become scarred and narrowed, leading to *dysphagia* and food sticking in the stricture. These can be stretched open by dilation procedure, but stricture formation is a sign that reflux treatment should be escalated.

Esophagitis. Inflammation of the esophagus, associated with reflux disease; biopsies will show many inflammatory cells.

Esophagogastroduodenoscopy (EGD). Examination of the esophagus, stomach, and duodenum (upper small bowel) usually performed by a gastroenterologist under heavy sedation. EGD is not the best way to examine the esophagus in reflux patients; see transnasal esophagoscopy.

Esophagus. The muscular swallowing tube that connects the throat and the stomach; the esophagus has two valves, one at the top where it attaches to the pharynx (throat) and one at the bottom where it attaches to the stomach.

Expiratory wheezing. Noisy breathing on exhalation characterized by restricted and prolonged exhalation, usually due to *asthma*.

Expiratory. Of or relating to exhalation, breathing out.

Extraesophageal reflux disease. Reflux that comes up above the esophagus into the throat; synonym for *respiratory reflux, airway reflux,* and *laryngopharyngeal reflux.*

Food and Drug Administration (FDA). Branch of government responsible for monitoring drug and food quality and safety. The GRAS ("generally regarded as safe") list is approved by the FDA. In 1973, the FDA decided that acid would be the main preservative for foods and beverages in bottles and cans, and acids make up 13 percent of the GRAS food additive list.

Fundoplication, laparoscopic fundoplication. Anti-reflux surgical procedure performed by freeing the dome (*fundus*) of the stomach and sewing (plicating) it around the esophagus to create a tight angle so that food in the stomach stays in the stomach, that is, prevents reflux. *Laparoscopic* means that the surgery is done with small instruments used through very small openings, i.e., there is no abdominal incision needed for this approach.

Gastric. Of or relating to the *stomach*.

Gastroenterologist, GI. An internal medicine specialist physician whose focus is the gastrointestinal tract.

Gastroesophageal reflux disease (GERD). This is the most commonly used medical term for *esophageal reflux*. Literally it means "stomach-esophagus back-flow disease."

GI. As above, *gastroenterologist*.

Globus, globus pharyngeus. A sensation of a lump in the throat, a common symptom of *airway reflux*; usually caused by UES (*upper esophageal sphincter*) dysfunction. Often children will describe that something is "stuck" in their throat and then may become anxious about eating and want only soft, pureed foods

Glottic stenosis. Scarring and narrowing at the level of the vocal cords decreasing space for airflow.

Granuloma. This is a benign growth that occurs in the larynx; associated with trauma and airway reflux.

H2-Antagonist (H2A). H2As are a class of acid-suppressive medications that are sometimes used to treat reflux. H2As are safe and do not need to be administered by a physician; they do not cause rebound hyperacidity and may be used on an as-needed basis. Common medications are listed shown on pages 172–173.

Heartburn. Chest pain related to reflux, usually after a large or fatty meal. It may be sometimes confused with a heart attack.

Hiatal hernia. An anatomic slippage of the lower esophageal sphincter above the diaphragm. By itself, a hiatal hernia is no a reason for anti-reflux surgery.

High-definition airway and esophageal ISFET pH monitoring. New, state-of-the-art reflux testing method invented by the author, Dr. Jamie Koufman. This technology is highly sensitive and specific for diagnosing respiratory reflux. (The ISFET chip, usually reserved for use in high-quality pH meters, has greatly increased the accuracy of testing for respiratory reflux.)

Hypopharynx. The lower part of the throat (pharynx); this includes the larynx (voice box), the piriform sinuses and the esophageal inlet (which form the uppermost opening into the *esophagus)*.

Idiopathic. A condition that occurs for an unknown reason or without a known cause.

Idiopathic pulmonary fibrosis. Progressive, chronic lung disease characterized by scarring in the lungs. This condition may be a complication of long-standing *airway reflux*.

Idiosyncratic trigger foods. Idiosyncratic means *something peculiar to an individual*. *Idiosyncratic foods* are foods that cause reflux in some people but not in others; an individual's *trigger foods* for reflux. Among the most common idiosyncratic trigger foods (across the population) are onions, garlic, tomatoes, nuts, wine, coffee, and chocolate.

Indigestion. Discomfort or difficulty digesting food, also called *dyspepsia*, may be associated with burping (eructation), gas, and *heartburn*.

Inspiratory. Of or relating to inhalation, breathing in.

Inspiratory stridor. Noisy breathing on inspiration. *Stridor* means noisy breathing.

Lap (laparoscopic) fundoplication. Anti-reflux surgical procedure performed by freeing up the dome *(fundus)* of the stomach and sewing (plicating) it around the esophagus to create a tight angle so that food in the stomach stays in the stomach, that is, prevents esophageal reflux. *Laparoscopic* refers to performing the *fundoplication* operation though multiple mini-incisions. (As of this writing, laparoscopic fundoplication is still the best surgical reflux treatment available.)

Laryngeal adductor reflex (LAR). Involuntary closure of the vocal cords due to irritation of the voice box that is controlled by the central nervous system.

Laryngeal nerves. The laryngeal (voice box) nerves that account for voice, cough, and airway protection during swallowing. The main vocal cord nerve is *the recurrent laryngeal nerve* and a second nerve, the *superior laryngeal nerve,* allows high-pitched voicing. All of these vocal cord (laryngeal) nerves are branches of the *vagus nerve.*

Laryngologist. A physician, usually an *otolaryngologist* (ENT doctor), who specializes in problems of the voice and throat, including *LPR, airway reflux*.

Laryngomalacia. Misshapen and increased floppiness of the cartilages that sit above the vocal folds during inspiration. The largest cartilage, or epiglottis, covers entrance into the airway during swallowing. Laryngomalacia can lead to very noisy breathing and reflux can worsen this condition.

Laryngopharyngeal reflux (LPR). Former name for *respiratory reflux*; LPR is still a commonly used term for the backflow of stomach contents into the throat, that is, the *laryngopharynx* (*larynx* and *pharynx*).

Laryngospasm. Laryngospasm in a type of *choking episode* in which the vocal cords clamp shut causing severe *inspiratory stridor*. By far the most common cause of laryngospasm is *airway reflux*.

Laryngotracheobronchitis (viral croup). Viral infection (croup) of the upper airway that causes swelling from the level of the vocal cords down to the trachea and bronchial lining of the lungs. It leads to a barky cough.

Larynx, laryngeal (voice box). Housing of the vocal cords, false vocal cords, and the epiglottis (cover). The larynx is responsible for three functions: (1) phonation (voice); (2) airway (it is through the larynx that air gets into the trachea/bronchi/lungs); and (3) sphincteric protection of the airway with swallowing. The sphincteric function of the larynx prevents *aspiration* by keeping foods or liquids out of the lungs.

Lifestyle factors. Time of eating, use of tobacco, too-tight belts or clothing, overconsumption of alcohol are all considered to be lifestyle factors that influence reflux. Of all the lifestyle factors, late (night) eating is the most commonly identified problem.

Lower esophageal sphincter (LES). The valve at the lower end of the esophagus where it joins the stomach. The LES opens to let food into the stomach and prevents *gastroesophageal reflux*. The anti-reflux surgical procedure, *laparoscopic fundoplication*, tightens the LES.

Motor nerve. An efferent—travelling from the brain—nerve that conveys impulses that cause muscular contraction.

Nasopharynx. The part of the upper throat behind the nose and above the palate.

Neurogenic cough. Nerve-caused cough; cough caused by *vagal neuropathy*, often associated with *post-viral vagal neuropathy*.

Neurogenic, neuropathic, neurogenic pain. Of or relating to a nerve; pain that is caused by a neuropathy or malfunctioning nerve.

Neuropathy. Sick nerve syndrome. Neuropathies may be caused by infections, such as *post-viral vagal neuropathy*, and by many other causes including trauma (injuries), autoimmune diseases, toxic exposures, and diseases such as diabetes, Lyme, and MS (multiple sclerosis). *Bell's palsy* and *post-viral vagal neuropathy* are common neuropathies.

Non-Pulmonary. Not of the lung(s), as in *non-pulmonary chronic cough*. Non-pulmonary implies that a problem in the lungs is *not* the cause of the chronic cough.

Nutrition. The processes by which an animal or plant takes in and utilizes food substances for sustenance. Food is necessary for human nutrition.

ORL (otorhinolaryngology, otolaryngology). An ENT (ear, nose, and throat) physician and surgeon who specializes in diseases of the ears, nose, and throat; the specialty is also called *otolaryngology—head and neck surgery*.

Oropharynx. That part of the throat behind the tongue and below the palate. The tonsils and the uvula are in the oropharynx.

Otolaryngologist. An ENT (ear, nose, and throat) physician and surgeon who specializes in diseases of the ears, nose, and throat; the specialty is also called *otolaryngology*—head and neck surgery.

Paralysis. Paralysis of a muscle or muscle group occurs when the nerve going to those muscle(s) is interrupted. The most common causes of *vocal cord paralysis* are *iatrogenic* (doctor-caused), e.g., thyroid cancer surgery and *post-viral vagal neuropathy*.

Paresis, paretic (see also *vocal cord paresis*). Partial paralysis, often as a consequence of viral infection, neck trauma or surgery.

Paroxysmal laryngospasm. Acute and severe reversal of the normal phasic movement of the vocal cords. With laryngospasm, the vocal cords close tightly during inspiration leading to airway obstruction and *inspiratory stridor*, almost a crowing sound. Typically, patients refer to laryngospasm as terrifying "choking episodes"; these laryngospasm attacks typically last minutes and are almost always caused by *airway reflux*. Laryngospasm is a frightening symptom. See also *laryngospasm*.

Pepsin assay. A test used to detect or measure *pepsin* (invented by Dr. Jamie Koufman).

Pepsin. The primary digestive enzyme of the stomach. Pepsin (and not acid) causes reflux-related tissue damage; it has also been implicated as the cause of esophageal and laryngeal cancer. (The author now has a non-invasive diagnostic test for reflux that detects pepsin in the saliva.)

pH, pH scale. The pH scale takes its name from the words *potential of hydrogen*. The pH scale is used to measure the acidity or alkalinity of a substance or solution. The pH scale ranges from 0 to 14, with pH 7 being neutral. Numbers above 7 indicate alkalinity and numbers below 7 indicate acidity. The scale is logarithmic, meaning that pH 2 is ten times more acidic than pH 3, and one-hundred times more acidic than pH 4. Stomach acid is typically pH 1–4, as are virtually all soft drinks today. Clinically, we know that consumption of beverages pH <4 is associated with reflux, particularly with *silent airway reflux*.

Pharyngeal. Of or relating to the *pharynx* (throat).

Pharynx, pharyngeal. The entire throat, from the back of the nose down to the lower end where it joins the *esophagus*. The uppermost portion is called the nasopharynx, and the lower portion is called the laryngopharynx, i.e., voice box/throat.

Pharynx. Medical term for the (entire) throat from the back of the nose (above) to the top of the *esophagus* (below).

pH-Balancing. pH-balancing is a way to reduce the impact of acidic foods by combining them with alkaline, as in having strawberries with low-fat milk (cow, almond, or soy).

pH-Monitoring. Reflux-testing method in which an ultra-thin device is swallowed and measures the pH in the throat and esophagus during a twenty-four-hour period. When a pH sensor is placed in the throat, this technology, using an ISFET chip, is the state of the art for evaluating *airway reflux*.

Post-nasal drip. The feeling that mucus is dripping into the throat from the back of the nose, and may be due to allergy, infection, toxic fumes, or reflux. It is one of the commonest symptoms of *airway reflux*.

PPI (proton pump inhibitor (PPI). See *proton pump inhibitor*.

Prokinetic, prokinetic agent. A class of medications that are for movement; usually used to treat *esophageal dysmotility* and poor esophageal valve function. The prokinetic agents include raglan, domperidone, erythromycin, and gabapentin.

Proton pump inhibitor (PPI). A class of acid-suppressive medications sometimes used to treat reflux. PPIs should be administered by a physician because they cause rebound hyperacidity when stopped abruptly. They should not be used on an as-needed basis. In addition, they should not be used long-term as they mask progression of disease, leading to complications of reflux, including esophageal cancer and precancer, lung, and sinus disease.

Pseudo-asthma, pseudo-asthmatics. A misdiagnosis of asthma. A condition, usually reactive airway disease caused by airway reflux, that is confused with asthma. People with pseudo-asthma, pseudo-asthmatics, usually have *inspiratory stridor* and not *expiratory wheezing*.

PUL (Pulmonologist). Chest physician, a medical doctor who specializes in problem of the lungs.

Pulmonary function tests (PFTs). A set of breathing tests designed to measure lung volumes and lung function; PFTs are useful in diagnosing *reactive airway disease*, *asthma*, and *COPD*.

Pulmonary. Of and relating to the lungs.

Pulmonologist (PUL). Chest physician, a medical doctor who specializes in problems of the lungs.

Pyloric Stenosis. Narrowing of the sphincter that leads from the stomach to the small intestines.

Ranitidine (Zantac). This acid-suppressive medication is an H2-antagonist. It is a safe and effective over-the-counter, anti-reflux medication suitable for use without a doctor's prescription.

Reactive airway disease, reactive airways. There are many different manifestations and diagnoses associated with the term *reactive airways*. In all cases, something triggers the airway to change its physiology (usually) in a way that produces distressing symptoms.

Recalcitrant. Refractory; resisting control; hard to deal with or manage.

Reflux esophagitis, esophagitis. Inflammation of the esophagus, associated with reflux disease; biopsies will show a lot of inflammatory cells.

Reflux finding score (RFS). The RFS is a validated outcomes instrument for quantifying the laryngeal findings of airway reflux.

Reflux laryngitis. See *laryngopharyngeal reflux* and *airway reflux*.

Reflux symptom index (RSI). The RSI is a validated outcomes instrument for quantifying the laryngeal symptoms of airway reflux; take the quiz on page 53.

Refluxate. A term for the actual material that refluxes; that is, the liquid mixture (composed of acid, stomach enzymes, and undigested food) that comes up.

Reflux-related cough. Cough that is caused by *airway reflux*.

Reflux-related reactive airway disease, reactive airway disease. Most reactive airway disease, with the exception of allergic rhinitis, is due to *airway reflux*.

Reflux-testing. A diagnostic method of documenting abnormal reflux in the airway and esophagus; the state of the art is *high-definition airway and esophageal ISFET pH monitoring* (see above).

Refractory. Hard or impossible to manage; resisting ordinary methods of treatment.

Regurgitation. The backflow of material from the *esophagus* or *stomach* into the mouth. People with regurgitation may complain of heartburn, indigestion, and a sour taste in the mouth.

Relapsing polychondritis. An idiopathic condition that causes persistent or recurrent inflammation of the cartilages of the body, often involving the ears, nose, larynx, and breathing passages such as the trachea and bronchi. If ineffectively treated, the disease can be fatal.

RFS. See *reflux finding score*.

RSI. See *reflux symptom index* above.

Sensory, **sensory nerve**. Pertaining to the senses or sensation, or a nerve that passes impulses from receptors toward or to the central nervous system (the brain).

Silent reflux. Connects *respiratory reflux and silent reflux*, that is, reflux that occurs without obvious symptoms (*heartburn* and *indigestion*). Within the context of this book, the term *silent reflux* is virtually synonymous with *silent respiratory reflux*. But theoretically, *silent airway reflux* may be differentiated from *silent esophageal reflux*.

Sinusitis. Inflammation and/or infection of the sinuses that may be caused by upper respiratory infection, allergy, or airway reflux.

Sleep apnea. A condition in which a person stops breathing during sleep; most cases are due to obesity, abnormal throat anatomy, and *airway reflux*. Snoring and generally noisy breathing are typical as well as daytime somnolence (sleepiness).

Stridor. Noisy (audible) breathing. Stridor may be inspiratory, expiratory, or both. *Inspiratory stridor* is associated with reflux, and expiratory stridor (*wheezing*) is associated with *asthma*.

Stroboscopy, videostroboscopy. A device used by *laryngologists* for studying the motion of the vocal cords, especially the vocal cord vibrations, by making the motion appear to slow down by periodically illuminating the vocal cords. Usually, stroboscopy is recorded on a video-system for slow-motion playback and analysis and shows vocal cord stiffness, scarring, or weakness (*paresis*).

Subglottic stenosis. Scarring and narrowing below the level of the vocal cords. Subglottic stenosis may be congenital and/or caused by respiratory reflux.

Tagamet (cimetidine). Acid suppressive medication.

TB. See *tuberculosis*.

TE (tracheoesophageal) Fistula. See *Tracheoesophageal fistula*.

TFL. See *transnasal laryngoscopy*.

Therapeutic trial. Deductive use of a specific treatment to make a specific diagnosis, that is, *empiric treatment* used as a diagnostic. If a treatment effectively alleviates a certain condition, it is assumed that the condition was the correct diagnosis.

TNE. See *transnasal esophagoscopy*.

Trachea. The main breathing tube that connects the bottom of the larynx (voice box) with the lungs.

Trachebronchial tumor. Benign or malignant tumor in the large airway, either *trachea* or *bronchi*.

Trachebronchial. Of or relating to the *trachea* and bronchial tubes.

Tracheoesophageal fistula (TE fistula). An opening between the esophagus and the trachea that causes continual contamination of the airway by whatever is swallowed, including saliva. The origin of a TE fistula may be congenital, traumatic, or *iatrogenic*.

Transnasal esophagoscopy (TNE). Examination of the esophagus (and upper stomach), usually performed by an otolaryngologist or gastroenterologist without sedation. TNE is the best way to examine the esophagus in reflux patients; transnasal esophagoscopy is preferred because it is a safer, more accurate, and less expensive examination.

Transnasal laryngoscopy, transnasal flexible laryngoscopy (TFL). This is the state-of-the-art throat/larynx (voice box) examination method. After spraying the nose with a topical numbing agent, an ultra-thin, flexible instrument (with a light and high-definition camera on the tip) is introduced through the nose and advanced into the upper throat. TFL is usually simultaneously performed with *videostroboscopy*, which allows closer examination of the vocal cords for *vocal cord paresis,* and it allows the examiner to compute the *reflux finding score.*

Transnasal. Literally, "through the nose," as in *transnasal esophagoscopy*. Usually an ultra-thin, flexible endoscope is used for all type of transnasal diagnostics and procedures.

Trigger foods. Foods (or beverages) that cause reflux and/or other symptoms such as throatburn. A *trigger food* can be any food, and there is great individual variation from person to person. Banana, for example, pH 5.7, is generally considered to be a good-for-reflux fruit; unfortunately, banana is a *trigger food* for 5 percent of people. The most common trigger foods are chocolate, coffee, wine, nuts, onion, tomato, garlic, and pepper.

Tuberculosis (TB). TB is still a significant cause of chronic cough in the Western world, and it should be ruled out by TB skin test and chest X-ray.

Turbinates. Three sets of bony shelves on the inside of the nose coming off of the sidewall of the nose, covered by mucous membrane that can swell or shrink. Turbinates make up the functioning organ of the nose to humidify, warm, and filter the air we breathe in.

Upper esophageal sphincter (UES). The valve at the upper end of the *esophagus* where it joins the *pharynx*. Actually the UES combines elements of both *pharyngeal* and *esophageal* anatomy. The UES is responsible for preventing *esophageal reflux* from entering the airway. When it fails, *airway reflux* occurs. The UES is also commonly responsible for *globus* symptoms.

Upper respiratory infection (URI). Generic name for a cold, the flu, or any infection that involves the nose and/or throat. URIs are believed to be responsible for *post-viral vagal neuropathies.*

Vagus (vagal) nerve (plural *vagi*). The vagus is the Xth cranial nerve, that is, its origins are in the brainstem and it exits the skull to traverse the neck running along the carotid sheath (with the carotid artery and the jugular vein). It lies right under the lining membranes of the throat making it vulnerable to viral infections. The vagus is the primary nerve of the entire aerodigestive (airway and digestive) tract, including the vocal cords, the cough reflux, the esophagus and the esophageal sphincters, and the stomach. It even sends branches to the heart, ear, and colon. Thus, *post-viral vagal neuropathy* may affect a host of vagally-mediated functions.

Vasomotor rhinitis. Runny/stuffy nose that results from dilation of the blood vessels inside the mucous membrane of the turbinates. There is increased activation and inflammation of the membranes. This is the diagnosis that applies to clinical allergies when no specific allergen can be identified

Videostroboscopy. *Videostroboscopy* is performed during the laryngeal examination by *transnasal flexible laryngoscopy* (TFL). Videostroboscopy is really two functions: (1) video-recording of the examination for subsequent frame-by-frame play back, and (2) stroboscopy for ultra-slow-motion analysis of vocal fold movement. A floppy vocal cord on stroboscopy, for example, is characteristic of subtle *vocal fold paresis* as seen in *post-viral vagal neuropathy*.

Vocal cord nerves. The laryngeal (voice box) nerves that account for voice, cough, and airway protection during swallowing. The main vocal cold nerve is the recurrent laryngeal nerve and a second nerve, the superior laryngeal nerve allows high-pitched voicing. All of these vocal cord (laryngeal) nerves are branches of the *vagus nerve*.

Vocal cord paralysis. Complete immobility of a vocal cord leading to *glottal closure symptoms*; see also *vocal cord paresis*, below.

Vocal cord paresis. Partial paralysis (weakness) leading to *glottal closure symptoms* such as vocal fatigue and effortful speaking, often due to *post-viral vagal neuropathy*.

Vocal fold. This is a synonym for *vocal cord*.

Voice disorders. Any problem or disorder that leads to *dysphonia* (hoarseness). Voice disorders encompass nerve-muscle problems such as *vocal cord paralysis* and *paresis*, brain-disorder problems such as Parkinsonism and spasmodic dysphonia, vocal cord growths such as nodules, polyps, and cancers, behavioral problems such as vocal abuse/misuse/overuse syndromes, and finally reflux.

Wheezing. Expiratory stridor, noisy breathing on exhalation, associated with asthma. Wheezing is also associated with prolongation of the expiratory phase of respiration.

Zantac. Brand name for an H2-antagonist acid-suppressive medication; see *ranitidine*.

REFERENCES

1. Koufman J, Stern J, Bauer M. *Dropping Acid: The Reflux Diet Cookbook & Cure.* New York: The Reflux Cookbooks; 2010.

2. Koufman J. Low-acid diet for recalcitrant laryngopharyngeal reflux: therapeutic benefits and their implications. *Ann Otol Rhinol Laryngol.* 2011; 120:281–287.

3. Koufman J. *The Chronic Cough Enigma: How to Recognize, Diagnose and Treat Neurogenic and Reflux-Related Cough.* New York: Katalitix Media; 2014.

4. Koufman J, Huang S, Gelb P. *Dr. Koufman's Acid Reflux Diet: With 111 All New Recipes Including Vegan & Gluten-Free: The Never-Need-to-Diet-Again Diet.* New York: Katalitix Media; 2015.

5. Wei J: *A Healthier Wei: Reclaiming Health for Misdiagnosed and Overmedicated Children.* New York: A Healthier Wei LLC; 2012.

6. Koufman. "Respiratory Reflux" (A Better Term for LPR). www.VoiceInstituteofNewYork.com, Blog post; 2016.

7. Pollan M. *The Omnivore's Dilemma: A Natural History of Four Meals.* New York: Penguin; 2007.

8. Davis, W. *Wheat Belly: Lose the Wheat, Lose the Weight, and Find Your Path Back to Health.* New York: Rodale; 2011.

9. Salatin J. *Folks, This Ain't Normal: A Farmer's Advice for Happier Hens, Healthier People, and a Better World.* Nashville: Center Street; 2012.

10. Lustig, R. *Fat Chance: Beating the Odds Against Sugar, Processed Food, Obesity, and Disease.* New York: Plume; 2012.

11. Perlmutter D, Loberg C. *Grain Brain: The Surprising Truth about Wheat, Carbs, and Sugar—Your Brain's Silent Killers.* New York: Little, Brown and Company; 2013.

12. Moss M. *Salt, Sugar, Fat.* New York: Random House; 2013.

13. Campbell TC, Campbell TM II. *The China Study: The Most Comprehensive Study of Nutrition Ever Conducted and the Startling Implications for Diet, Weight Loss, and Long-Term Health.* Dallas: BenBella Books; 2016.

14. Andersen K, Kuhn K. *What the Health.* Documentary film; 2017.

15. *Food Inc* (on Netflix and Amazon).

16. *Forks Over Knives* (on Netflix and Amazon).

17. Wei J. TEDx Talk: Milk and Cookie Disease. Available at https://www.youtube.com/watch?v=R2C6bBNWGp0

18. Greger M, Stone. *How Not to Die: Discover the Foods Scientifically Proven to Prevent and Reverse Disease.* New York: Flatiron Books; 2015.

19. Wolchover N. Can mountain dew really dissolve a mouse carcass? *Scientific American*; January 5, 2012. https://www.scientificamerican.com/article/can-mountain-dew-really-dissolve

20. Little FB, Koufman JA, Kohut RI, Marshal RB. Effect of gastric acid on the pathogenesis of subglottic stenosis. *Ann of Otol Rhinol Laryngol* 1985; 94:516–519.

21. Wiener GJ, Copper JB, Wu WC, Koufman JA, Richter JE, Castell DO. Is hoarseness an atypical manifestation of gastroesophogeal reflux? *Gastroenterology.* 1986; 90:A1691.

22. Koufman JA, Wiener GJ, Wu WC, Castell DO. Reflux laryngitis and its sequelae: The diagnostic role of 24-hour pH monitoring. *J Voice.* 1988; 2:78–89.

23. Weiner GJ, Koufman JA, Wu WC, et al. Chronic hoarseness secondary to gastroesophageal reflux disease: Documentation with 24-H ambulatory pH monitoring. *Amer J Gastroenterol.* 1989; 84:12.

24. Koufman JA. The otolaryngologic manifestations of gastroesophageal reflux disease (GERD): A clinical investigation of 225 patients using ambulatory 24-hour pH monitoring and an experimental investigation of the role of acid and pepsin in the development of laryngeal injury. *Laryngoscope.* 1991;101 (Suppl. 53):1–78.

25. Koufman JA. Aerodigestive manifestations of gastroesophageal reflux. What we don't yet know. *Chest.* 1993; 104:1321–1322.

26. Koufman JA. Methods and compositions for the diagnosis of extraesophageal reflux. United States Patent 5,879,897; 1996.

27. Koufman JA, Sataloff RT, Toohill R. Laryngopharyngeal reflux: Consensus report. *J Voice.* 1996; 10:215–216.

28. Loughlin CJ, Koufman JA. Paroxysmal laryngospasm secondary to gastroesophageal reflux. *Laryngoscope.* 1996; 106:1502–1505.

29. Loughlin CJ, Koufman JA, Averill DB, et al. Acid-induced laryngospasm in a canine model. *Laryngoscope.* 1996; 106:1506–1509.

30. Koufman JA, Burke AJ. The etiology and pathogenesis of laryngeal carcinoma. *Oto Clin N A.* 1997; 30:1–19.

31. Little JP, Matthews BL, Glock MS, Koufman JA, et al. Extraesophageal pediatric reflux: 24-hour double-probe pH monitoring of 222 children. *Ann Otol Rhinol Laryngol Suppl.* 1997; 169: 1–16.

32. Matthews BL, Little JP, McGuirt Jr. WF, Koufman JA. Reflux in infants with laryngomalacia: Results of 24-hour double-probe pH monitoring. *Otolaryngol Head Neck Surg.* 1999; 120:860–864.

33. Koufman JA, Amin M, Panetti M. Prevalence of reflux in 113 consecutive patients with laryngeal and voice disorders. *Otolaryngol Head Neck Surg.* 2000; 123:385–388.

34. Duke SG, Postma GN, McGuirt Jr. et al. Laryngospasm and diaphragmatic arrest in the immature canine after laryngeal acid exposure: A possible model for sudden infant death syndrome (SIDS). *Ann Otol Rhinol Laryngol.* 2001; 110:729–733.

35. Belafsky PC, Postma GN, Koufman JA. Laryngopharyngeal reflux symptoms improve before changes in physical findings. *Laryngoscope.* 2001; 111: 979–981.

36. Belafsky PC, Postma GN, Daniels E, Koufman JA. Transnasal esophagoscopy. *Otolaryngol Head Neck Surg.* 2001; 125:588–589.

37. Reulbach TR, Belafsky PC, Blalock PD, Koufman JA, Postma GN. Occult laryngeal pathology in a community-based cohort. *Otolaryngol Head Neck Surg.* 2001; 124:448–450.

38. Postma GN, Tomek MS, Belafsky PC, Koufman JA. Esophageal motor function in laryngopharyngeal reflux is superior to that of classic gastroesophageal reflux disease. *Ann Otol Rhinol Laryngol.* 2001; 110:1114–1116.

39. Belafsky PC, Postma GN, Koufman JA. The validity and reliability of the reflux finding score (RFS). *Laryngoscope.* 2001; 111:1313–1317.

40. Amin MR, Koufman JA. Vagal neuropathy after upper respiratory infection: a viral etiology? *Am J Otolaryngol.* 2001; 22:251–256.

41. Amin MR, Postma GN, Johnson P, Digges N, Koufman JA. Proton pump inhibitor resistance in the treatment of laryngopharyngeal reflux. *Otolaryngol Head Neck Surg.* 2001; 125:374–378.

42. Johnson PE, Koufman JA, Nowak LJ, et al. Ambulatory 24-hour double probe pH monitoring: The importance of manometry. *Laryngoscope.* 2001; 111:1970–1975.

43. Smoak BR, Koufman JA. Effects of gum chewing on pharyngeal and esophageal pH. *Ann Otol Rhinol Laryngol.* 2001;110:1117–1119.

44. Axford SE, Sharp S, Ross PE, et al. Cell biology of laryngeal epithelial defenses in health and disease: Preliminary studies. *Ann Otol Rhinol Laryngol.* 2001; 110:1099–1108.

45. Koufman JA, Belafsky PC, Daniel E, Bach KK, Postma GN. Prevalence of esophagitis in patients with pH-documented laryngopharyngeal reflux. *Laryngoscope.* 2002; 112:1606–1609.

46. Belafsky PC, Postma GN, Koufman JA. Transnasal esophagoscopy (TNE). *Otolaryngol Head Neck Surg.* 2001; 125: 588–589.

47. Koufman JA. Laryngopharyngeal reflux is different from classic gastroesophageal reflux disease. *Ear Nose Throat J.* 2002; 81:7–9 2002.

48. Belafsky PC, Postma GN, Koufman JA. Validity and reliability of the reflux symptom index (RSI). *J Voice.* 2002; 16:274–7.

49. Belafsky PC, Postma GN, Koufman JA. Subglottic edema (pseudosulcus) as a manifestation of laryngopharyngeal reflux. *Otolaryngol Head Neck Surg.* 2002; 126:649–652.

50. Koufman JA. Laryngopharyngeal reflux is different from classic gastroesophageal reflux disease. *Ear Nose Throat J.* 2002; 81:7–9.

51. Koufman JA. Laryngopharyngeal reflux 2002: A new paradigm of airway disease. *Ear Nose Throat J.* 2002; 81(9 Suppl 2) 2406.

52. Cohen JT, Bach KK, Postma GN, Koufman JA. Clinical manifestations of laryngopharyngeal reflux. *Ear Nose Throat J.* 2002; 81:14–23.

53. Koufman JA, Aviv JE, Casiano RR, Shaw GY. Laryngopharyngeal reflux: Position statement of the Committee on Speech, Voice, and Swallowing Disorders of the American Academy of Otolaryngology—Head and Neck Surgery. *Otolaryngol Head Neck Surg.* 2002; 127:32–35.

54. Johnston N, Bulmer D, Gill GA, et al. Cell biology of laryngeal epithelial defenses in health and disease: Further studies. *Ann Otol Rhinol Laryngol.* 2003; 112:481–491.

55. Westcott CJ, Hopkins MB, Bach KK, et al. Fundoplication for laryngopharyngeal reflux. *J American College of Surgeons.* 2004; 199:23–30.

56. Halum SL, Postma GN, Johnston C, et al. Patients with isolated laryngopharyngeal reflux are not obese. *Laryngoscope.* 2005; 115:1042–5.

57. Postma GN, Cohen JT, Belafsky PC, et al. Transnasal esophagoscopy revisited (over 700 consecutive cases). *Laryngoscope.* 2005; 115:321–3.

58. Johnston N, Knight J, Dettmar PW, et al. Pepsin and carbonic anhydrase isoenzyme III as diagnostic markers for laryngopharyngeal reflux disease. *Laryngoscope*. 2004; 114:2129–34.

59. Knight J, Lively MO, Johnston N, et al. Sensitive pepsin immunoassay for detection of laryngopharyngeal reflux. *Laryngoscope*. 2005; 115:1473–8.

60. Gill GA, Johnston N, Buda A, et al. Laryngeal epithelial defenses against laryngopharyngeal reflux (LPR): Investigations of pepsin, carbonic anhydrase III, pepsin, and the inflammatory response. *Ann Otol Rhinol Laryngol*. 2005; 114:913–21.

61. Johnston N, Dettmar PW, Lively MO, Koufman JA. Effect of pepsin on laryngeal stress protein (Sep70, Sep53, and Hsp70) response: Role in laryngopharyngeal reflux disease. *Ann Otol Rhinol Laryngol*. 2006; 115:47–58.

62. Johnston N, Dettmar PW, Bishwokarma B, et al. Activity/stability of human pepsin: Implications for reflux attributed laryngeal disease. *Laryngoscope*. 2007; 117:1036–9.

63. Amin MR, Postma GN, Setzen M, Koufman JA. Transnasal esophagoscopy: A position statement from the American Broncho-Esophagological Association. *Otolaryngol Head Neck Surg*. 2008; 138:411–3.

64. Koufman J, Block. Differential Diagnosis of Paradoxical Vocal Fold Movement. *Am J Speech Lang Pathol*. 2008; 17:327–34.

65. Koufman JA, Johnston N. Potential Benefits of pH 8.8 Alkaline Drinking Water as an Adjunct in the Treatment of Reflux Disease. *Ann Otol Rhinol Laryngol*. 2012; 121:431–34.

66. Koufman J. Opinions: Obama's acid reflux may help others receive proper diagnosis and treatment. *Washington Post*. December 8, 2014.

67. Koufman J. Opinion: The dangers of eating late at night. *New York Times*. October 25, 2014.

68. Koufman J. Opinion: The specialists' stranglehold on medicine. *New York Times*. June 3, 2017.

69. Cicala M, Emerenziani S, Luca MP, et al. Proton pump inhibitor resistance, the real challenge in gastro-esophageal reflux disease. *World J Gastroenterol*. 2013; 19: 6529–6535. Published online 2013 Oct 21. doi: 10.3748/wjg.v19.i39.6529.

70. Childhood Obesity Facts: Prevalence of Childhood Obesity in the United States. https://www.cdc.gov/obesity/data/childhood.html. Centers for Disease Control and Prevention. April 10, 2017.

71. Fryar CD, Carroll M.D., Ogden CL. Prevalence of overweight and obesity among children and adolescents in the United States, 1963–1965 through 2011–2012. Atlanta, GA: National Center for Health Statistics; 2014.

72. Ogden CL, Carroll M.D., Lawman HG, et al. Prevalence of overweight and obesity among children and adolescents in the United States, 1988–1994 through 2013–2014. *JAMA*. 2016; 315:2292–9.

73. Cheung PC, Cunningham SA, Naryan KMV, Kramer MR. Childhood obesity incidence in the United States: A systematic review. *Child Obes*. 2016; 12:1–11.

74. Daniels SR, Hassinik SG. The role of the pediatrician in primary prevention of obesity. *Pediatrics*. 2015; 136275–92.

75. Jacobson BC, Somers SC, Fuchs CS, et al. Body-mass index and symptoms of gastroesophageal reflux in women. *NEJM*. 2006; 354: 2340–2348.

76. Lang JE, Hossain J, Holbrook JT et al. Gastro-oesophageal reflux and worse asthma control in obese children: a case of symptom misattribution? *Thorax*. 2016; 71:238–46.

77. Hassink, S. Updates recommendations on obesity prevention: It's never too early to begin living a healthy lifestyle. *American Academy of Pediatrics*. June 29, 2015.

78. Karp H. *The Happiest Baby on the Block: The New Way to Calm Crying and Help Your Newborn Baby Sleep Longer*. 2nd Rev. Ed. New York (NY): Bantam; 2015.

79. Hegar B, Boediarso A, Firmansyah A, et al. Investigation of regurgitation and other symptoms of gastroesophageal reflux in Indonesian infants. *World J Gastroenterol*. 2004; 10:1795–97.

80. Miyazawa R, Tomomasa T, Kaneko H, et al. Prevalence of gastro-esophageal reflux-related symptoms in Japanese infants. *Pediatr Int*. 2002; 44:513–16.

81. Nelson SP, Chen EH, Syniar GM, et al. Prevalence of symptoms of gastroesophageal reflux during infancy. A pediatric practice-based survey. Pediatric Practice Research Group. *Arch Pediatr Adolesc Med*. 1997; 151:69–572.

82. Martin AJ, Pratt N, Kennedy JD, et al. Natural history and familial relationships of infant spilling to 9 years of age. *Pediatrics*. 2002; 109:1061–1067.

83. Vandenplas Y, Rudolph CD, Di Lorenzo C, et al. Pediatric gastroesophageal reflux clinical practice guidelines: joint recommendations of the North American Society for Pediatric Gastroenterology, Hepatology, and

Nutrition (NASPGHAN) and the European Society for Pediatric Gastroenterology, Hepatology and Nutrition (ESPGHAN). *J Pediatr Gastroenterol Nutr.*
2009; 49:498–547.

84. McMahon B. The continuing enigma of pyloric stenosis of infancy: A
review. *Epidemiology.* 2006; 17:195–201.

85. Hill, DL. Baby's first bowel movements. Available at HealthyChildren.org.
American Academy of Pediatrics. Nov 21, 2015.

86. Shalaby TM, Orenstein SR. Efficacy of telephone teaching of conservative
therapy for infants with symptomatic gastroesophageal reflux referred by pediatricians to pediatric gastroenterologists. *J Pediatr.* 2003; 142: 57–61.

87. Sharma S, Kolahdooz F, Butler L, et al. Assessing dietary intake among
infants and toddlers 0–24 months of age in Baltimore, Maryland, USA. *Nutr
J.* 2013; 26:52.

88. American Academy of Pediatrics announces new safe sleep recommendations to protect against SIDS, Sleep-Related Infant Deaths. Oct. 24, 2016.
Available at https://www.aap.org/en-us/about-the-aap/aap-press-room/pages/
american-academy-of-pediatrics-announces-new-safe-sleep-recommendations-
to-protect-against-sids.aspx.

89. Res-Q-Wedge. Available at https://www.resqwedge.com.

90. U.S. Food and Drug Administration. Do Not Use Infant Sleep Positioners
Due to the Risk of Suffocation. Available at https://www.fda.gov/ForCon-
sumers/ConsumerUpdates/ucm227575.htm.

91. Grimes CA, 1 Szymlek-Gay EA, Nicklas TA. Beverage Consumption
among U.S. Children Aged 0–24 Months: National Health and Nutrition
Examination Survey (NHANES) Nutrients 2017, 9, 264; doi:10.3390/nu
9030264.

92. Miles G, Siega-Riz SAM. Trends in Food and Beverage Consumption
Among Infants and Toddlers: 2005–2012. Pediatrics. May 2017. See at
http://pediatrics.aappublications.org/content/early/2017/04/27/peds.2016–3
290.

93. Fruit Juice and Your Child's Diet. HealthyChildren.org. Available at
https://www.healthychildren.org/English/healthy-living/nutrition/Pages/Fruit-
Juice-and-Your-Childs-Diet.aspx.

94. Gajanan M. Babies Should Not Drink Fruit Juice, Doctors Group Says
Time, May 22, 2017. Available at http://time.com/4788078/fruit-juice-guide-
lines-babies-aap.

95. Health concerns about dairy products. Physicians Committee for Responsible Medicine. Available at http://www.pcrm.org/health/diets/vegdiets/health-concerns-about-dairy-products.

96. Clyne PS, Kulczycki A. Human breast milk contains bovine IgG. Relationship to infant colic? *Pediatrics*. 1991; 87:439–44.

97. Ornish D, Brown SE, Scherwitz LW, *et al.* Can lifestyle changes reverse coronary heart disease? The lifestyle heart trial. *Lancet*. 1990; 336:129–33.

98. Thorning TK, Raben A, Tholstrup T, et al. Milk and dairy products: good or bad for human health? An assessment of the totality of scientific evidence. *Food Nutr Res*. Nov 22 2016;60. (This study was sponsored by the dairy industry.)

99. Hendrickson, K. Carbonic acid in beverages. Livestrong.com. Oct 3, 2017. Available at http://www.livestrong.com/article/547245-carbonic-acid-in-beverages.

100. TH Chan. Soft drinks and disease. Harvard School of Public Health. Available at https://www.hsph.harvard.edu/nutritionsource/healthy-drinks/soft-drinks-and-disease.

101. Kamala, T. The awful truth about diet soda and weight gain according to science. *Forbes*. Sept 8, 2016. Available at https://www.forbes.com/sites/quora/2016/09/08/the-awful-truth-about-diet-soda-and-weight-gain-according-to-science/#347f589d462f).

102. Shaw, G. Soda and osteoporosis: Is there a connection? WebMD. Webmd.com. Feb 1, 2007. Available at http://www.webmd.com/osteoporosis/features/soda-osteoporosis#1.

103. Teenagers and Coffee: Caffeine and your teen. Coffee Home Direct. 2011. Available at http://www.coffeehomedirect.com/coffee-and-teenagers. Retrieved Oct 21, 2017.

104. Mullen, M and Shield JE. Water: How much do children need? Eat Right: Academy of Nutrition and Dietetics. Available at http://www.eatright.org/resource/fitness/sports-and-performance/hydrate-right/water-go-with-the-flow. May 2 2017.

105. World corn production by country 2016/17 (1 in 1,000 metric tons) *Statista*. 2017. Available at https://www.statista.com/statistics/254292/global-corn-production-by-country retrieved October 21 2017.

106. Lonoir M, Serre F, Cantin L, Ahmed SH. Intense sweetness surpasses cocaine reward. *PLoS ONE*. 2007; 2: e698, 2007. Available at https://www.ncbi.nlm.nih.gov/pmc/articles/PMC1931610.

107. Bentley J. USDA. U.S. per capita availability of red meat, poultry, and fish lowest since 1983. Economic Research Service. Available at https://www.ers.usda.gov. February 6, 2017.

108. Swearingen, D. Eating before competitions. Central Washington University. Available at https://www.cwu.edu/sports-nutrition/eating-competition. Retrieved October 21, 2017.

109. Kovar I, Selstam U, Catterton W, et al. Laryngeal chemoreceptors in newborn lambs: respiratory and swallowing response to salts, acids and sugars. *Pediatr Res.* 1979; 13:1144–1149.

110. Tieder JS, Bonkowsky JL, Etzel RA, et al. Brief resolved unexplained events (formerly apparent life-threatening events) and evaluation of lower-risk infants: Executive summary. *Pediatrics.* 2016; 137:e20160591.

111. Allergy testing in children and infants. American College of Allergy, Asthma & Immunology (ACAAI) organization (2014). Available at http://acaai.org/allergies/allergy-treatment/allergy-testing/allergy-testing-children-and-infants. Retrieved Oct 21 2017.

112. Sicherer S, Wood RA. Section on allergy and immunology. Allergy testing in childhood: Using allergen-specific IgE Tests. *Pediatrics.* 2012; 129:193–7.

113. American Thoracic Society Patient Information Series. *Am J Respir Crit Care Med.* 2014; Vol. 189, P5–P6. Available at https://www.thoracic.org/patients/patient-resources/resources/pulmonary-function-testing-children.pdf.

114. Northway WH, Rosan RC, Porter DY. Pulmonary disease following respiratory therapy for hyaline membrane disease: bronchopulmonary dysplasia. *N Eng J Med.* 1967; 276:357–68.

115. Jobe AH, Bancalari E. Bronchopulmonary dysplasia. *Am J Resp Crit Care Med.* 2001; 163:1723–9.

116. Nobile S, Noviello C, Cobellis G, et al. Are infants with bronchopulmonary dysplasia prone to gastroesophageal reflux? a prospective observational study with esophageal ph-impedance monitoring. *J Pediatr.* 2015; 167:279–85.

117. Diagnosed with cystic fibrosis. Cystic Fibrosis Foundation. Available at https://www.cff.org/What-is-CF/Diagnosed-With-Cystic-Fibrosis.

118. Robinson NB, DiMango E. Prevalence of gastroesophageal reflux in cystic fibrosis and implications for lung disease. *Annals of the American Thoracic Society.* 2014; 11: 964–68.

119. Brodzicki J, Trawinska-Bartnicka M, Korzon M. Frequency, consequences and pharmacological treatment of gastroesophageal reflux in children with cystic fibrosis. *Medical science monitor: international medical journal of experimental and clinical research.* 2002; 8(7) Cr529–37.

120. Boesch, RP and Acton, JD. Outcomes of fundoplication in children with cystic fibrosis. *J Pediatr Surg.* 2007; 42 (8)1341–1344.

121. Smith LP, Chewaproug L, Spergel JM and Zur KB. Otolaryngologists may not be doing enough to diagnose pediatric eosinophilic esophagitis. *Int J Pediatri otorhinolaryngol.* 2009; 73:1554–7.

122. Langer J. Intestinal rotation abnormalities and midgut volvulus. *Surg Clin N Am.* 2017; 97:147–159.

123. TE Fistula and Esophageal Atresia foundation website: http://www.eatef.org.

124. Coleman B, Adzick NS, Crombleholme TM, et al. Fetal therapy: state of the art. *J Ultrasound Med.* 2002; 21:1257–88.

125. Huoh K, Messner A. Cricopharyngeal achalasia in children: indications for treatment and management options. *Curr Opin Otolaryngol Head Neck Surg.* 2013; 21:576–80.

126. Romano C, van Wynckel M, Hulst J. et al. European society for pediatric gastroenterology, hepatology and nutrition guidelines for the evaluation and treatment of gastrointestinal and nutritional complications in children with neurological impairment. *JPGN.* 2017; 65:242–64.

127. Moyer MW. Don't be fooled into thinking Welch's fruit snacks are any healthier than candy. Slate.com. Sept 25, 2015.

128. Sugarscience. Sugar in plain sight: sugar is in 74% of packaged foods. University of California San Francisco. Available at http://sugarscience .ucsf.edu/hidden-in-plain-sight/#.We4mZVtSz3i.

GENERAL INDEX

Acid, stomach
  acid reflux and, 5, 16
  defined, 15
Acid reflux
  causes, scientific summary of, 7
  childhood obesity and, 10–11
  children two to twelve, 37–51
  defined, 16
  development of, 8–10
  diagnosis, xiii
  as great masquerader, xi
  kid-friendly conversation, 14–18
  as link between diet and disease, 3–13
  as missing link, xii
  newborn to age two, 19–36
  quizzes for determining, 11–13
  symptoms, 16–17
  teens, 52–58
  trigger foods, 74
Acids
  dietary, as problem, 3
  food acidity. See pH
  properties of, 4
  use in foods, 4–5
Airway and lung problems, 177–89. See
    also Allergies; Asthma
  about: combined gastrointestinal and
    airway problems, 192–95;
    overview of, 177–79; potentially
    serious signs/symptoms and,
    177–79
  aspiration, 186–87
  brief resolved unexplained event
    (BRUE), 182
  bronchopulmonary dysplasia (BPD),
    188
  congenital diaphragmatic hernia
    (CDH), 194
  cricopharyngeal (CP) achalasia, 194–
    95
  cystic fibrosis (CF), 188–89
  foreign bodies in airway, 183–84
  glottic and subglottic stenosis, 187

laryngomalacia, 178, 179–80
laryngospasm, 180–81
pneumonia (recurrent), 192
sudden infant death syndrome
    (SIDS), 182
tracheoesophageal fistula (TEF) and
    esophageal atresia (EF), 192–94
Alginates, 172
Aliases
  allergy, 46–47
  asthma, 39
  babies, 21
  children, 40–47
  chronic cough, 40, 45
  congestion, 44–45
  croup, 45–46
  noisy breathing, 42–44
Alkaline diet. See Low-acid diet
Alkaline water, 8
Alkalines (bases), 4
Allergies. See also Asthma
  alias, 46–47
  babies and, 22–23
  children and, 46–47
  symptoms and testing, 184–86
American Academy of Pediatrics (AAP),
    23, 33
American diet, 3
Antacids, 172, 173
Anti-reflux medications. See Medications
    (reflux)
Anti-reflux surgery, xvii, 27, 174
Aspiration, 186–87
Asthma
  alias, 39, 40–41
  allergies, symptoms, and testing, 184–
    86
  diagnosis, 42
  medical test to diagnose, 41
  underlying cause of inflammation
    and, 41
Athletes, eating before practice, 79

INDEX OF INGREDIENTS IN RECIPES

Fennel, 126
Figs, 114
Fish and seafood. *See* Arctic char; Clams; Halibut; Salmon and salmon roe; Shrimp
Flour, 98, 99, 100, 130, 131, 161
Flour tortillas, 97

Garbanzo beans (chickpeas), 115, 158
Garlic, (121–23), 125, (141–43), 155
Ginger (fresh and ground), 92, 100, 104, 106, 128, 134–35, 138, 144, 146, 147, (153–55), 159, 162, 163, 168, 169
Ginger juice, 168
Grapes, 93
Grape seed oil, 99, 100, 109, 126, 128, 129
Green beans, 115, 125, 134–35, 142–43, 163

Halibut, 148
Honey, 92, 100, 114, 147, 160, 168, 169
Honeydew melon, 93, 95, 159
Horseradish, 109

Iceberg lettuce, 163

Kale, 114, 118
Kidney beans, 115

Lemon, 137, 139
Lemon juice, 114, 169
Lemon zest, 115, 118, 169
Lettuce, 149, 163. *See also* Mesclun greens; Spring mix (greens)

Maple syrup, 97, 98, 114, 161, 166, 167
Marjoram, 117
Melons. *See* Cantaloupe; Honeydew melon; Watermelon
Mesclun greens, 112–13
Milk, 92, 98, 105, 130, 146–47, 169. *See also* Almond milk; Soy milk
Mirin, 115, 118, 138
Miso, 138

Molasses (blackstrap), 130
Mushrooms, 105, 116, 134–35, 140, 144, 146, 148, 154
Mustard greens, 132
Mustard powder, 115, 117

Noodles/pasta, 150, 154
Nutmeg, 98, 110

Oat flour, 98
Oats, 97, 166
Oil. *See* Grape seed oil
Olive oil, 97, 107, 108, 112, (114–18), (121–32), (134–39), (141–55), (159–61), 163, 164
Olives, 117, 129, 149
Onions, 122, 134–35
Orange juice, 112–13, 141
Oregano, 107, 108, 112–13, (115–17), 126
Oyster sauce, 163

Palm sugar, 99, 154
Paprika, 108–9, 121
Parmesan cheese. *See* Cheese, Parmesan
Parsley, 104, (105–9), 115, 116, 122, 128, 129, 159
Parsnips, 128, 142–43
Pasta/noodles, 150, 154
Peaches, 94
Pears, 95, 113, 169
Peas, 107, 108, 145
Pepper, bell, 134–35
Pineapple, 159
Pine nuts, 163
Pistachios, 167
Popcorn, 164
Pork, tenderloins, 146–47. *See also* Prosciutto
Potatoes, 104, 108, 128
Prosciutto, 102, 142–43, 148, 158
Pumpkin purée, 100
Pumpkin seeds, 118

Quinoa flakes, 100
Quinoa flour, 100

Radicchio, 112, 116
Radishes, 112
Raisins, 112–13
Raspberries, 93
Rice, 127, 132, 140, (144–47)
Rice vinegar, 115
Rice wine. *See* Wine, rice
Romaine lettuce, 149
Rosemary, 107, 108, 113, 116, 139,
    146–47

Salmon and salmon roe, 96, 137, 138,
    139, 145, 162–63
Sea bass, 153
Seaweed stock, 108, 128, 154
Seeds. *See specific seed types*
Sesame oil, 115, 141, 144, 147, 153
Sesame seeds, 113, 117, 158
Sherry vinegar, 115
Shrimp, 150
Sour cream, 98, 102, 103
Soy milk, 97, 99, 161
Soy sauce/tamari, 115, 134, 141, 146,
    147, 153, 154, 155, 160, 162, 163
Spinach, 93, 113, 132
Split peas, 107
Spring mix (greens), 114
Squash. *See* Butternut squash; Zucchini
Star anise, 146, 147
Strawberries, 93
Sugar, 146, 155. *See also* Agave sugar;
    Brown sugar; Palm sugar
Sweet potatoes, 122, 125, 128, 160

Tamari. *See* Soy sauce/tamari
Tea, black, 162
Thyme, 102, 105, 107, 108, (115–17),
    140, 158, 160
Tofu, 132, 134
Tomatoes, 114
Tortillas (flour), 97

Turkey (ground), 146, 149, 163
Turmeric, 127

Vanilla extract, 97, 99, 169
Vegetable stock, 103, 104, 107, 108,
    127, 128, 140, 148, 151, 154

Walnuts, 112
Watermelon, 169
White beans, 107
Whole-wheat flour, 131
Wine
    port, 110
    rice, 128, 141, (146–48), 153, 154,
        155
    white, 107, 129

Yeast (dry), 130, 131
Yogurt, 76, 92

Zucchini, 142–43, 150

ABOUT THE AUTHORS

Dr. Jamie Koufman, one of the world's leading authorities on the diagnosis and treatment of acid reflux, is responsible for coining the terms "laryngopharyngeal reflux," "silent reflux," "airway reflux," and "respiratory reflux." She is the Founder and Director of the Voice Institute of New York and Clinical Professor of Otolaryngology at the New York Eye & Ear Infirmary of the Mt. Sinai Medical System. Dr. Koufman is a *New York Times* bestselling co-author of *Dropping Acid: The Reflux Diet Cookbook & Cure*, the first book to offer refluxers an understanding of reflux that emphasized low-acid diet and lifestyle changes to achieve a natural cure. She is also the author of *The Chronic Cough Enigma* and *Dr. Koufman's Acid Reflux Diet*.

Dr. Julie L. Wei is Professor of Otolaryngology—Head and Neck Surgery at the University of Central Florida School of Medicine and is Surgeon-in-Chief of Nemours Children's Hospital. She is also the Division Chief of Pediatric Otolaryngology. For many years, Dr. Wei has observed the significant relationship between dietary habits and children's health, which resulted in publication of her book, *A Healthier Wei—Reclaim Health for Misdiagnosed and Overmedicated Children*.

Dr. Karen Zur is the Director of the Pediatric Voice Program and Associate Director of the Center for Pediatric Airway Disorders at Children's Hospital of Philadelphia (CHOP). As a mother of two and a surgeon with a busy aerodigestive practice, she sees the impact and importance of healthy eating as well as the role that reflux plays on a child's ear, nose, throat, voice, and airway problems.

ACKNOWLEDGMENTS

The authors would like to thank the people who added to this book's content and helped improve it in many ways. Special thanks to the editors and readers who helped us develop, shape, and refine this book: Ian Howland, Michele Matrisciani, Tom Golodik, Latasha Taylor, Catherine Koufman, and Dr. Maria Mascarenhas.

A great-kids thanks to Dr. Jamie's grandchildren who helped with the "Kid-Friendly Reflux Conversation": Holden, Annie, J.D., and Lula.

Thanks and love to Dr. Julie's 11-year-old daughter Claire, who taught her that good eating, sleeping, and life habits are critical in raising a healthy child. She is also grateful to her husband David, who has tirelessly supported her journey and commitment to increase public awareness on the importance of healthy diet and lifestyle to prevent symptoms that lead to misdiagnosis and overmedication in children.

Much love and thanks to Dr. Zur's 8-year-old twin daughters who helped perform the pH-testing on all of the baby food and formulas available in Center City Philadelphia. She is thankful to her husband, Robert Biron, who has been a constant voice of reason and love.

Thanks to the many chefs whose recipes are contained in our "Recipes for Reflux Repair" section: Marc Bauer, Jordan Stern, Sonia Huang, and Philip Gelb, as well as the coauthors of this book, each of whom contributed recipes.

Finally, the authors are deeply grateful to the parents and their children who were courageous enough to take a chance and follow our recommendations for changing their children's eating habits to overcome acid reflux.